BREATHE EASY
An Asthmatic's Guide
to Clear Air

ALSO BY STANLEY REICHMAN
Instant Fitness for Total Health

BREATHE EASY

An Asthmatic's Guide
to Clear Air

Stanley Reichman, M.D., F.A.C.P.

THOMAS Y. CROWELL COMPANY
Established 1834, New York

LIBRARY OF CONGRESS CATALOGING IN PUBLICATION DATA

Reichman, Stanley.
  Breathe easy.

  Includes index.
  1. Asthma. I. Title.
RC591.R44   616.2'3   77-4109
ISBN 0-690-01480-5

10   9   8   7   6   5   4   3   2   1

TO MY DAUGHTER, DEBBI,

in the hope that her breathing will always
be free and her living will
always be easy.

Acknowledgment

It is with deep gratitude that I wish to thank the many individuals who helped me gather data and who encouraged the preparation of this manuscript. To Drs. J. Levine and B. Meyers an especial thanks is due. And to my family and my dear wife, I am particularly appreciative for their continued patience.

Contents

PART II.   UNDERSTANDING YOUR ASTHMA

PART III.   WHAT CAN BE DONE AND WHAT YOU
SHOULD EXPECT

Preface

Medicine has made enormous achievements during this century. Many contagious diseases have been virtually conquered, and people are living longer and in greater comfort.

Good health through preventive medicine that's truly preventive is a major goal today. That people believe this is an achievable goal is reflected in the current national demand for more primary health care and better personalized medical care. These demands require a new examination of the relationship between the physician and the patient.

In many cases, perhaps even most, this relationship is not what it could be. As a patient, your welfare requires the best possible communication and understanding between you and your doctor. It also requires your recognition that the physician is often only your adviser. He can tell you what needs to be done, but only you can do it.

If you suffer from asthma, your situation might be likened to your being alone in a small rowboat in a rough sea, taking directions about the safest way to shore from a professional (the doctor) standing on a cliff. The professional can warn about rocks and shoals, but it's up to you to row.

When you tell a doctor your symptoms, you are really asking for help. When the doctor begins his examination, he is really saying, "I'll try."

Thus a contract between patient and doctor begins. But the contract is incomplete unless the patient also makes a contract with himself—a contract designed to achieve specific health goals.

The overweight person can obtain a diet from his physician; the diabetic, a diet and an insulin prescription; and the person with high blood pressure, a pill to reduce his hypertension. But unless each individual develops a program for himself which he weaves into his daily living, the desired results are not achieved. This is especially true in the case of the asthmatic. The physician can prescribe, but the final results are in the hands of the patient.

The purpose of this book is to make the asthmatic more aware of personal needs, of the causes of asthma, of preventive measures, of options for treatment, and to encourage him or her to set personal goals for prevention and control. It is my hope, as a physician, that each asthmatic will design a contract based on specific needs and objectives.

Explore your asthma. Learn to control it. Take a little time and find what pathways lead you most quickly to clear air—to full, normal breathing. While your doctor advises and sets your course, you are the one who must row the boat. In the ultimate, only you can make sure you will breathe free and easy.

What Is Happening and
Why It Is Happening

1

The First Steps

"I'm going to die!"

If you have ever had an acute asthmatic attack, the conviction that you can't survive almost inevitably has swept over you. Shoulders hunched, head thrust forward, chest bellowed out, desperation fills you as you struggle to push the air out of your lungs and to acquire new air. Often, within moments, sweat pours from your body, trickles over your scalp. Your back becomes hard as wood. Your chest feels totally constricted. If you are wearing anything close-fitting around your neck—even a turtleneck or a tie or a light necklace—you want to tear it off. You wheeze, gasp, even moan. You know a drink of water would help, but in the acute attack you feel it is impossible to drink water. You think it won't go down; that, somehow, it could even worsen your breathing difficulties.

Friends and relatives watching an asthmatic in an acute attack are likely to share the conviction that the asthmatic is about to die. Terrified, they may watch the attack worsen. Sometimes the asthmatic is unable to walk, unable to stand. Eyeballs roll. The skin turns blue.

3

I've never forgotten the first asthmatic attack of Jessica P., a pretty Californian, mother of two babies, one a year old, the other, three. Jessica came from a sheltered, upper-class family and a home in an area distant from city pollution. Her husband, an engineer, brought her to New York where he was studying for his doctorate, acutely aware that New York's smells, its dirt, its hot summers and cold winters upset her, and that their tiny, servantless apartment disturbed her. Now, watching Jessica in the throes of the asthmatic attack, he was frantic and was almost as much trouble to me as Jessica, who had told him, gaspingly, that she was dying.

"What will happen to my babies when I die? Promise me you'll take them home to California to my mother. She will take care of them."

Her fright washed over her in waves during the time that it took to finally break the asthma attack and restore her to near-normal breathing. Asthma was a totally new and terrifying experience to Jessica. No one in her family had ever had asthma. She had never seen anyone with an asthmatic attack. Now, struggling for the breath she had always taken for granted, in her mind she saw herself dead, her husband remarried, and her children neglected by the new wife. Her fright and tears aggravated the attack.

And, of course, sometimes asthmatics have died during an asthmatic attack—deaths that might have been prevented if the asthmatic had understood his asthma, had developed and followed a program to control and prevent the asthmatic attack, and had learned what to do when an attack occurred.

YOUR INVOLVEMENT

Asthma can be controlled.

For many, asthma can be brought to remission.

For almost everyone, easy breathing is an achievable goal.

But only you, the asthmatic, can achieve it. And you can do that only when you understand the causes of your asthma. Many asthmatics in this country treat their problem lightly by simply using an over-the-counter drug to aid their breathing. But that is a dangerous course. Every asthmatic should have a physician as advisor. In addition, there are things that you need to know about asthma, that you need to know about yourself. This book will help you obtain that knowledge. It will help you get the best possible assistance from a skillful physician who agrees that the patient has the right to be fully informed about his treatment and his options, and that, in the final analysis, it is the patient who controls his destiny. And it could well be that, from the knowledge you gain from this book, you will be able to eliminate those factors from your life which have been causing your asthma.

The important thing to know is that asthma can be controlled and that, unless you do control it, you are courting serious complications. Commonly, chronic asthma leads to a decrease in the elasticity of the lungs, to bronchitis, and to other pulmonary afflictions. Emphysema, unnecessary complications during surgery, or even heart failure can occur.

Some asthmatics have had the disease since infancy. Others develop asthma as adults, frequently as a result of an infection, as in the case of Jessica, whose attack was preceded by a severe and lingering cold. Allergy is the usual cause in infants and children, although many adults, who have been bothered by allergies for years, seem suddenly to develop asthma, a situation often triggered by an infection.

It is this group of "spontaneous" adult asthmatics who, experiencing their first attacks, are likely to think that death is at hand. In Jessica's case, it was a relatively simple matter to begin treatment to make her comfortable. Educating her and her husband about asthma was not so simple.

Sometimes a "cold," or upper respiratory infection, is misleading. Arnold T., a busy, 47-year-old attorney, is an example. He called me because he had developed a "chest cold," which seemed to get better, then worsened. He saw a doctor near his home who gave him an antibiotic. Again Arnold seemed to improve. He resumed his smoking habit, which he had foregone during the worst period of his "cold," and immediately found himself coughing again and suffering from shortness of breath. When he called me, he complained: "I just can't get rid of this bloody chest cold. It's over a month now."

When I saw him, he had wheezes and was distinctly short of breath on mild effort. His cough was not productive of enough mucus for me to feel that he had a lingering bronchitis, and he had not had an acute asthmatic attack. When his chest X-ray proved normal, I told him he was having a mild asthmatic attack.

"Don't be silly," he said. "I haven't had asthma since I was a kid."

"Why didn't you mention having had asthma?" I asked.

"I forgot," he replied.

It was a little easier to explain to Arnold what was happening than to Jessica, but still I was surprised at how little he knew about this disease that had plagued his childhood.

I've found that patients often do have an extensive understanding of their asthma. They can almost predict attacks. They use their medications wisely. But, whenever I've asked detailed questions, I've learned that there was more they could have done, if they had known they had additional options. The problem then is to find out what each individual needs to know, and then to teach what the options are. As a doctor and a teacher, this is a challenge—and it's a basic reason I'm writing this book.

Asthma has both physical and psychological roots. To bring it under control, you must first decide to seek all help possible and, second, you must examine your life style and those attitudes which could interfere with a program of prevention and control.

THE CONTRACT

I believe that good health should be possible for everyone— reasonably good health, at least. However, as a doctor, I know the help I can offer depends, for its effectiveness, upon your goals. Since you are reading this book, I assume that one of your goals is to know more about asthma, and that another is to bring your asthma under control. To help you achieve these goals, I urge you to make a contract with yourself to be successful in overcoming your asthmatic handicap. This contract, which you will sign in order to help you acquire better health, will probably be less elaborate than the buy-sell contract for an automobile or a TV set, but it will be a lot more important.

This "Personal Asthma Contract" may be written on a single page, or run several pages. It's up to you to design your own contract. Its scope will depend upon *your* condition and *your* objectives.

If you suffer only occasionally from asthma and mildly at that, you may have few objectives. If you have severe, chronic asthma, your objectives will be much more comprehensive, and your contract may have many dimensions. But in either case, your contract will deal with three basic goals:

1. an understanding of asthma in general and specifically of yourself and why *you* have asthma;

2. the creation of an effective, personal program of prevention;

3. the establishment of methods of control should attacks occur.

While this may sound complicated, if you approach it step by step, I am certain you will not find it difficult, and I'm confident it will pay off in the end.

WHY SHOULD I LEARN?

You may ask: "Why should I learn about asthma when I can just go to my doctor and get medicine?"

Of course, you can and should go to your doctor and get medicine and secure relief. But to do *only* that is the short-term, old-fashioned system of illness-cure or illness-control. "Prevent my illness!" is the contemporary cry and prevention calls for the patient's *understanding* of causes, and *commitment* to the goals of good health.

By learning more about asthma, you can understand the specific causes of your asthma; know the situations or environmental conditions that are likely to cause attacks, in order to eliminate or minimize them; know what to do when an attack threatens or occurs; become aware of other hazards; and come to know that your health is really in your hands.

Summed up, the best answer to "Why should I learn about asthma?" is to reduce the severity of attacks that occur, increasingly prevent attacks, or terminate them yourself, quickly. The longer an asthmatic attack lasts, the harder it is to terminate.

WHAT SHOULD I LEARN?

"What should I learn?" you may ask.

The answer to that will vary with the individual. It will relate to both the severity of the asthma and the individual's desire for knowledge. No one expects you to become a professional, but it is essential that you take time to gain all relevant information. Every asthmatic—and every interested parent, wife, or husband of an asthmatic—should understand the basic causes of asthma, and the specific causes in the individual who is the asthmatic.

Some of you may want to learn *everything*, whether or not it's relevant to *your* asthma. Others may want to learn only those things that help specifically. For instance, if your asthma is not caused by allergic reactions, you may not think it necessary to learn about allergies; however, you should be aware that sometimes the cause *is* an allergy and the asthmatic doesn't know it. If psychological factors cause your asthma, then you need to learn what those factors are, how to recognize and prevent them, or otherwise deal with them. By the time you have completed this book, you should be knowledgeable about asthma and will long since have answered for yourself that question "What should I learn?"

WHAT SHOULD I ASK?

While I am always asked specific questions about a patient's asthma or about specific complaints, patients or their families also inevitably ask me certain general questions. These questions, shown in Table 1, summarize the kinds of information people most want.

These questions are grouped under four basic questions that I believe you should ask whenever you go to a physician, no matter what is wrong. I call them the "What, Why, What, What" questions. They are:

1. *"What is happening?"* This means, "What is taking place within?" If you are an asthmatic, the question means: "What is happening in my lungs?"

2. *"Why is it happening?"* This means, "What are the causes?"

3. *"What can we do?"* This means, "What kind of treatment is available?" and "Are there tests I should take?"

4. *"What can I expect?"* This means, "What is the prognosis? What will, or could, happen in the future?"

Take a notebook or clip some paper together. Call these pages your worksheets. Head the first page: GENERAL QUESTIONS. Now begin to list all the general questions you've ever had about asthma.

TABLE 1. General Questions

What Is Happening?
   a) What happens during an attack?
   b) What makes it hard to breathe?
   c) What happens to the lungs?
   d) What causes the cough?
   e) What causes the mucus?

Why Is It Happening?
   a) Is there a single cause or many causes?
   b) Does asthma run in families?
   c) Is it always allergy?
   d) Is there something special that can start an attack?
   e) Can "nerves" be a factor?

What Can We Do?
   a) How can we stop attacks?
   b) What tests do I need?
   c) What medicine is the best?
   d) Can I prevent attacks?

What Can I Expect?
   a) Will it go away?
   b) What complications can occur?

Refer to Table 1. Under the heading, "Why Is It Happening?" look the questions over. If you know all the answers, you might be able to go right to the second section of this book. But first, think about these questions awhile, for they may suggest others that I have not listed. On the page labeled GENERAL QUESTIONS, try to classify the questions as I have done, adding new ones to those in the table. Questions under the headings, "What Can We Do?" and "What Can I Expect?" will be answered in later chapters.

I would like to make one other suggestion now. Take a second page for a worksheet. Make a heading titled: SPECIFIC QUESTIONS ABOUT MYSELF. List any questions about yourself that occur to you so that you can refer to them later. Some of these may be important. If the answers are not in this book, you may need to consult your doctor to find out if there is something special about your asthma. Take the time to fill out your worksheets. If it will help you overcome your asthmatic handicap, your time will be well spent. As you gather information, keep a goal of asthma control in mind, together with advice I first learned as a medical student: "Act as if it were impossible to fail."

At this point, all you need to know is that it *is* possible to control asthma. To start you on your way to clear air and easy breathing, let me suggest how to write the contract with yourself that I have mentioned.

Take a blank sheet of paper. Title it: MY PERSONAL ASTHMA CONTRACT. Put your name and date at the top of the sheet and then, as a first heading, write at the left margin your first goal: "Gain Understanding of Asthma." To the right, put a heading marked, "Date Completed." Underneath, put two subheadings, relating to asthma in general and *your* asthma. Your contact should look like the one on the facing page.

After your contract has been fully completed, you should write at the bottom "I commit myself to controlling my asthma," and sign your name.

MY PERSONAL ASTHMA CONTRACT

Name _____   Date _____

Goal I. Gain Understanding of Asthma   Date Completed

  1) General Knowledge   _____

  2) Specific Knowledge About Myself   _____

2

What Is Happening?

Every doctor wants to cure all his patients. Sometimes we fantasize and see ourselves realizing that dream. In reality, however, we know that all we can do is apply our knowledge and our intuition to do three things:

1. try to diagnose the patient's problem;
2. try to determine the causes of the problem, which may have many roots and factors;
3. prescribe a remedy or remedies, or a program.

When a patient becomes ill, the patient and doctor alike expect and hope that the doctor's prescription will produce a cure. Sometimes patients or their relatives become infuriated when the doctor's prescription falls short of that.

One Monday morning, an angry young mother, 27, arrived at my hospital with her blond, 6-year-old son, Andy, in tow. I happened to pass through the crowded waiting room as she walked in. Ignoring the others, she blazed out: "Your lung pills don't work! Andy had a terrible night!"

When we see an asthmatic having an attack, we don't make him wait his turn. The manifestations of the acute attack are so distressing that every doctor wants to end them as quickly as possible. With a quick explanation to the waiting patients, "an asthmatic," Andy, with his irate mother, was ushered into an examination room. The nurse quickly prepared him for the examination. When the pediatrician put his stethoscope on Andy's chest and listened, he heard rattles and slight wheezes. As treatment was given to open up the bronchial passages, the pediatrician and I discussed the problem. Then, while the pediatrician went on to another patient, I turned to Andy's mother.

"Asthma is not a simple disease," I explained. "It is a complex of symptoms with a variety of causes—sometimes multiple causes—and treatment that controls asthma in one case may not in another. The fact that Andy had an attack during the night does not mean that the pills he is taking are not the best thing for him. There may have been a special factor that caused last night's attack—a factor that does not normally exist. Has he had any sign of a cold, for instance?"

Before she could answer, Andy's little hand touched my arm. I turned to him. It was obvious that his breathing was much easier.

"What is asthma?" he asked.

I studied his bright, intelligent face.

"What do you think it is?" I returned.

"Something that makes it hard for me to breathe," he said. "Air goes in me, but it doesn't want to come out."

"That's a very good explanation of asthma," I said. "Asthma is caused by many things—by different things in different people—and sometimes when you have an asthmatic attack your breathing sounds different than on other occasions. Isn't that true?"

Andy nodded. "Sometimes I wheeze," he said, "and sometimes I don't."

"That's right. And some asthmatics don't ever wheeze, and some people who wheeze don't have asthma."

As I spoke I drew a sketch on a pad. Then, as I continued to draw, I explained what happens in an asthmatic attack. It occurred to me at that time that there are many people who have never studied biology in school. And many who *have* studied biology have forgotten a great deal about the lungs. For this reason it is important to review what actually happens when we breathe. In this way we will better understand the asthmatic attack, for even though Andy and others improve after treatment, understanding is the beginning of prevention.

LUNG STRUCTURE AND FUNCTION

Anatomy. The lungs lie within the chest. Besides the lungs, the four principal structures in the chest are the heart; the esophagus—the tube through which food passes from the mouth to the stomach; the aorta—the great artery through which the blood is pumped from the heart to all parts of the body; and the vena cava—the great vein through which blood eventually returns from all parts of the body to the heart.

The lungs are spongy in texture because of the millions of air sacs they contain. They are liberally supplied with blood vessels and have a double circulation. One circulation, the bronchial arteries and veins, supplies blood to nourish and maintain both the right and left lungs. The second consists of the pulmonary arteries and veins. This circulation collects oxygen from the air sacs and also unloads carbon dioxide into the air sacs so that it may be exhaled.

The lungs do not work by themselves. Air enters the lungs because of the expansion of the chest in inspiration. As you breathe in or inspire, you expand the chest in all directions. Your diaphragm descends, increasing the vertical diameter of the chest (see Figure 1). The muscles between each pair of ribs contract, thereby raising the ribs. The movement of the upper ribs increases the diameter of the chest from back to front by pushing the sternum forward. Enlargement of the chest creates a vacuum so that air is sucked into the lungs, causing them to expand. The lungs are highly elastic so that during expiration—when you breathe out—they recoil. Elasticity of the lungs is an important factor in easy breathing.

During extreme exertion, or in forced or difficult breathing, muscles of your neck and shoulder may also be involved in breathing, in order to increase air passage.

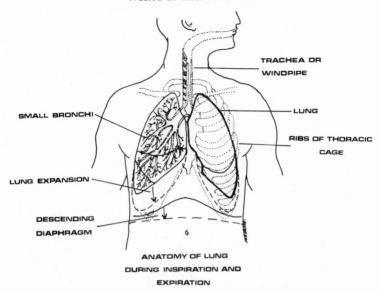

TRACHEA OR
WINDPIPE

SMALL BRONCHI

LUNG

RIBS OF THORACIC
CAGE

LUNG EXPANSION

DESCENDING
DIAPHRAGM

ANATOMY OF LUNG
DURING INSPIRATION AND
EXPIRATION

FIGURE 1.
As the diaphragms descend, the thoracic cage enlarges. Air enters the trachea passing through the large and then small bronchial tubes. The lungs expand as the air reaches the smaller air sacs as shown by the dotted lines (see text).

The muscles of the walls of the abdomen also are involved, exerting a controlling influence on the lower ribs. By expanding when you breathe in, they assist the descent of the diaphragm. The action of the abdominal muscles is most marked in forced expiration, as in certain breathing exercises that will be found in the Appendix, and in blowing up a balloon, or playing a wind instrument, such as a tuba or a clarinet. This is important because breathing exercises can be used by asthmatics to increase air flow. In this respect the diaphragm is especially important.

The diaphragm divides the chest or thorax from the abdomen. It is a dome-shaped sheet of muscular and fibrous tissue with ligaments and tendons. The diaphragm is attached to the inner surfaces of the lower ribs and spine and to the lower end of the sternum. It contains openings for passage of the esophagus, the vena cava, the aorta, and for certain glandular vessels and nerves. Except for these openings, the diaphragm completely separates the chest structures from the abdominal contents.

Breathing. When you breathe, air normally enters the nose, which filters large dust particles and warms very cold air; it then passes through the back of the throat to the windpipe or trachea, which ultimately divides into two branches. These branches, one on each side, are called bronchi. Each bronchus divides into many branches, called bronchial tubes, which in turn divide into smaller branches, the bronchioles.

Picture your breathing apparatus as an upside-down tree with hollow trunk and hollow branches. The windpipe can be compared to the tree trunk; the bronchial tubes to the larger branches, and the bronchioles to the smaller branches or twigs. The outside of each hollow branch is made up of elastic tissue. The inside of the branches is a soft, moist, mucous membrane.

The bronchioles connect to the lung tissue or air sacs, called alveoli. Think of the lungs as a balloon. Air goes in and out of the neck of a balloon easily, which becomes large as the air enters. Now picture your lungs as having millions of tiny, tiny balloons. What happens, of course, is that the air travels through the bronchial tubes and fills the "balloons"—the air sacs of the lungs. Oxygen from the air then diffuses into capillaries which line the air sacs. In this manner, oxygen enters the bloodstream, where it is taken up by the red blood cells. At the same time, carbon dioxide enters the air sacs (see Figure 2).

The term *respiration* signifies the process of breathing in and out to exchange new air for "used" air. This goes on continually and is a condition required for existence of every living cell. When we breathe in, we take in oxygen and a tiny bit of carbon dioxide. When we breathe out, we exhale quite a lot less oxygen and a great deal more carbon dioxide. This breathing cycle of inhalation-exhalation occurs normally in adults at rest at the rate of about twelve to sixteen times per minute. The cycle may be more rapid with children.

AIR SACS OF THE LUNG

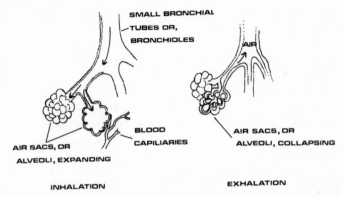

FIGURE 2.
As air fills the air sacs or alveoli from the bronchial tubes, they expand. As air is exhaled the air sacs collapse, leaving a small amount of residual air.

Depending upon the purity of the atmosphere, the air you inhale may contain about twenty-one percent of oxygen and less than four-tenths of one percent of carbon dioxide. The air you exhale will contain about sixteen percent oxygen and the carbon dioxide content will have increased to almost four and one-half percent. This gaseous exchange takes place in the alveoli at a very rapid rate over an internal lung surface that may be as much as 1,000 square feet. The bloodstream—that two-way street—is coursing through the linings of the alveoli at a rate of about nine pints per minute, taking in about 300 cubic centimeters of oxygen and, simultaneously, liberating about 250 cubic centimeters of carbon dioxide. That's the rate when you're resting. When you exercise, the blood flows more rapidly and the gaseous exchange process speeds up. During vigorous exercise, the blood flow and gaseous exchange may increase as much as four to six times over the "at rest" rate.

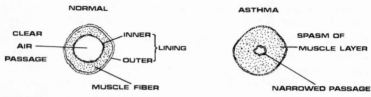

FIGURE 3.
A normal bronchiole and a bronchiole in spasm. Note the narrowed passage on the right.

THE ASTHMATIC ATTACK

In an asthmatic attack, spasm of the elastic covering of the bronchial tubes occurs, squeezing the tubes and making them smaller. The diaphragm descends, expecting to suck in air through the bronchioles but the spasm has contracted them so there is hardly room for any air to enter. It's like trying to suck in air through a straw (see Figure 3).

Although the cause of asthmatic attacks in children and adults may occur for different reasons, there are two separate physiological mechanisms which can induce spasm. The first mechanism causes narrowing of the bronchial tubes through a reflex action of the autonomic nervous system, following stimulation by various irritants. The second mechanism produces bronchospasm following a direct chemical reaction on the lining cells of the bronchial tubes. As an example of the first mechanism, nervous stimulation may occur after an emotional reaction. An example of the second would be local cellular reactions occurring as an allergic response to a substance.

THE AUTONOMIC NERVOUS SYSTEM

While there is a voluntary nervous system which controls your muscles for voluntary movements, there is also an involuntary nervous system. The bronchial tubes are lined by the involuntary nerves. There are two types of involuntary nerves which supply the bronchial tubes. One set, called *sympathetic* nerves, causes relaxation, or dilation, of the bronchial tubes. The other set causes constriction and belongs to the *parasympathetic* system. Both sets of nerves are called autonomic nerves because they work automatically; that is, they are not controlled by voluntary or thinking mechanisms. All of the heart and many respiratory responses are automatic in nature. This is probably a good thing. If we had to remember to breathe or cause our heart to beat, we could forget and this would be disastrous.

The sympathetic nerves are controlled by certain chemicals. Adrenalin is one. A substance produced by the center of the adrenal gland, adrenalin enables the body to cope with emergency situations. Adrenalin increases the heart rate and blood pressure, transfers blood from the skin and stomach to skeletal muscles, and inhibits digestion. When it is injected into the bloodstream, the effect is a powerful but short-lived stimulation of the whole sympathetic nervous system, causing, among other things, dilation of the bronchial tubes.

THE CELLULAR REACTION AND HEREDITY

While various irritants, perhaps notably the emotions, may cause autonomic reflex action and asthmatic attacks for many, there is another mechanism that can cause an attack. As I have already mentioned, a spasm can begin because of a chemical reaction in the lining cells of the inner membranes of the bronchial tubes. Certain cells are stimulated, or provoked, by a variety of either allergic or non-allergic factors to liberate spasm-producing compounds. The details of some very complicated reactions are becoming available through current research. These reactions are important because they will affect the development of new treatments, and increase the understanding of the role of heredity. Recent information suggests that there may be a permanent or inherited background abnormality in patients in whom these reactions take place. To say this another way, there may be individuals who have an increased sensitivity to various kinds of provoking factors.

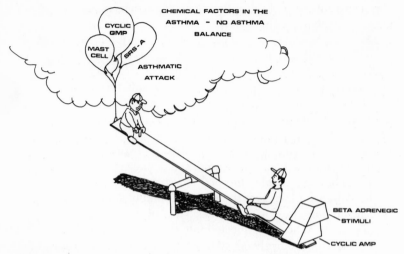

FIGURE 4.
The greater weight on the balance produced when cyclic AMP is more abundant, perhaps helped by beta adrenegic stimuli is shown with clear air resulting. The lesser weight, symbolized by the balloons when mast cells release SRS-A or other factors such as histamine or prostaglandins which favor increased cyclic GMP, results in decreased air or asthma.

Some believe there is a biochemical key to this sensitivity. The biochemical key is a balance within the cells between two complicated, cyclic, chemical substances which are abbreviated with the initials AMP and GMP. These cyclic chemicals work in a seesaw fashion. Those elements which favor an excess of GMP will have a particularly adverse effect and produce response from specific cells, called *mast* cells, which are likely to cause bronchial spasm. In Figure 4, notice that when the seesaw balances in favor of the AMP, no asthma takes place, but that when the balance favors the GMP, the "mast cell" produces chemical compounds which may initiate an asthma attack. These compounds include histamine, SRS-A, and some prostaglandins; the presence or absence of beta adrenergic stimuli act to potentiate or inhibit the different actions of the compounds.

But whatever the basic cause, this chemical concept is important because of an interaction with the autonomic nervous system. Thus, regardless of where the mechanism begins which initiates bronchospasm, drugs which induce a greater balance of cyclic AMP, or which stimulate the sympathetic nervous system to dilate a narrowed bronchial tree, will benefit the asthmatic.

If this seems very complicated, let me assure you that you are right. Because I have tried to simplify the cellular and autonomic nervous system reactions, I have omitted many scientific details which link both systems and make it impossible to say that one mechanism never occurs without the other. The following points are worth emphasizing:

Some people are born with a greater susceptibility to develop chemical reactions which favor asthma. Commonly these are allergic individuals.

The allergic asthmatic attack does not necessarily result from an increase in autonomic nervous response.

But the allergic person may respond to an adrenalin injection which acts through the sympathetic nerves.

The allergic person probably inherits an allergic factor from a member of his family. Other members of the family may not seem to be allergic, however. Parents who have allergies may or may not have allergic children. For purposes of treatment, it is important to distinguish allergic individuals.

Allergic asthmatics may respond to some medications which affect the cellular factors.

Whatever the cause, the asthmatic attack is characterized by an obstructive process in the small bronchial tubes. This obstruction varies in intensity and depends upon how much spasm is present. The term we doctors use is bronchospasm. The more spasm, the more difficulty there is in breathing.

BRONCHOSPASM

Wheezing is caused by bronchospasm. If you would try to suck in air through a narrow tube, you would find the air tends to make a whistling noise. However, if the obstruction and narrowing are great, there may be no wheezing since there is too little space for air to pass.

In mild asthma, the squeaks and groans and whistles may be audible only when the asthmatic takes a deep breath or when one listens with a stethoscope. An asthmatic may not even be aware of any shortness of breath until he exerts himself, and, between attacks, the asthmatic may feel and appear entirely normal.

When the attack occurs, however, the degree of obstruction is the important thing. Two things may happen in addition to spasm. The first is that the cells lining the bronchial membranes may become swollen. The term edema is used for swelling. Second, the lining cells, shocked and reacting to the spasm, may trigger secretions. Sometimes the secretions are watery, producing a thin, clear, or slightly white, sputum.

If the reaction persists, mucus may form. As air travels in and out of the narrowed passages, it passes over the mucus which may fur-

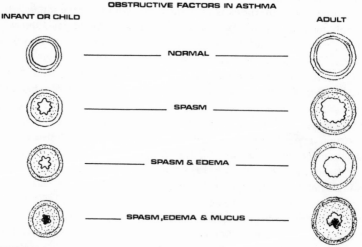

FIGURE 5.
Besides spasm and edema, the size of the bronchial tubes is a factor in obstruction. As the child becomes older and the bronchial tubes grow, the chances of complete obstruction become more remote.

ther block the passages. Besides wheezing, rasping or gurgling sounds, called rales, may become audible. Sometimes the tubes can be blocked completely, particularly in the case of a baby.

In an infant the bronchial tubes are normally narrow, so that there is less room for air and more likelihood of blockage. As a child grows older, the tubes become much wider so that complete obstruction is unlikely (see Figure 5).

The first objective of treatment is to lessen the spasm—to cause the elastic covering of the bronchial tubes to relax or even dilate so that mucus becomes loosened and can be coughed up.

SECRETIONS

Sputum is the secretion from the respiratory mucous glands. It comes in many types and colors. Sometimes it's white and watery but then turns sticky. Sometimes it contains solid-appearing yellow pellets. Sometimes it appears thicker, or even green. Sputum, generally, is related to duration of attack and the presence or absence of infection, and sometimes is an indication of an external condition.

For instance, Jackie, one of my young patients, had his parents exceedingly worried because the sputum he coughed up sometimes contained blackish specks. It took very little detective work to discover that Jackie and his parents lived in an old New York brownstone where the landlord used coal for heating. In Jackie's case, the dark sputum represented excess dust in the air resulting from stoking the coal furnace.

The role of infection in asthma will be explored in detail later. At this point, you should know that what is often thought to be a "cold" or "bronchitis" or a "night cough" may really be an asthmatic attack with or without a superimposed cold or upper respiratory infection.

When bacteria, or viruses, invade the membranes of the bronchial tree, the sputum often becomes yellow or green in color.

The most severe abnormalities occur when mucus plugs develop in the bronchial tubes and completely obstruct the passage. These plugs develop because, as the water content diminishes, the mucus becomes thick and firm (see Figure 6). Certain types of treatment for an asthmatic are aimed at liquefying the mucus.

THE RESPIRATORY TREE

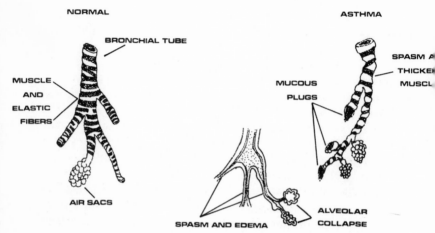

FIGURE 6.
As the attack occurs, the mucous glands in the bronchial wall are stimulated and may produce plugs of mucus which can further block a passage already constricted by muscle spasm and edema.

If mucus plugs develop in localized areas and a sufficient amount of oxygen can cross the other remaining lung membranes, no problems will develop, although localized segments of the lung can become infected. When the lung becomes infected, it is called pneumonia.

Later you will be asked to review your life history, to see if you can identify patterns of attacks. This may help you characterize the kind of asthma you have. For now, the important thing to remember is the concept of obstruction. If you can't get air into your lungs, you can't get oxygen into your bloodstream, and special centers which register blood oxygen content, called chemoreceptors, send a message to your brain to make you breathe harder.

Up to this point, I have sought to simplify my description of asthma. The alterations of function, which take place when abnormalities exist—what doctors call pathologic physiology—are complicated. Bear with me for just a little longer while I define chemoreceptors and aspects of breathing.

CHEMORECEPTORS

Chemoreceptors affect the respiratory, or breathing, centers in the brain. These centers, called carotid bodies, are regulated by decreasing oxygen and increasing carbon dioxide in the blood, and are located at a branch of the body's main blood vessel known as the aorta. Excess of oxygen decreases the stimulation from these carotid bodies to the brain and slows the need to breathe. Increase or accumulation of carbon dioxide does the reverse. Thus the chemoreceptors are message centers. Any sensation of shortness of breath is directly related to their activity. When you run up a hill and use up a lot of oxygen, your overbreathing is a result of their stimulation. Similarly when the lungs are not functioning properly, such as during asthmatic attacks, your need for oxygen or excess of carbon dioxide is being signaled to your brain to change your respiration.

ALTERED LUNG FUNCTION IN ASTHMATICS

Breathing, or inspiration and expiration, is the moving of air back and forth through the respiratory passage. The medical term used to describe this process is pulmonary ventilation. Pulmonary ventilation changes dramatically during an asthmatic attack. Normally, the bronchial tubes become widened during inspiration, and narrowed during expiration. During an asthmatic attack, however, the normal passage of the bronchial tubes is greatly distorted by spasm. When edema is present, it becomes even more difficult for air to leave the lungs. As a result, a positive force is required to squeeze out air.

Remember, the lungs have a certain amount of elasticity which permits them to recoil during expiration. This recoil helps dispose of air, making the breathing process a passive one. In the asthmatic, however, the powerful muscles of breathing, which are mostly used to inhale, must be used to force air out of the lungs. When this

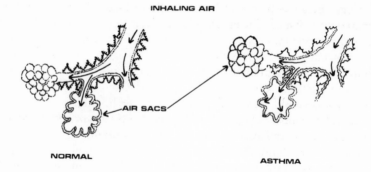

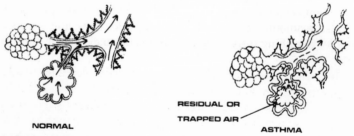

FIGURE 7.
When the bronchial tubes are narrowed during an asthmatic attack, or the spring-like attachments of the bronchial airways are lost (as in emphysema), recoil of the lungs is reduced. Though the act of breathing allows air to enter the lungs, the trapped or residual air seen on the right results from both the narrowed bronchial tube and loss of elastic recoil as the condition becomes protracted.

happens, the phase of breathing out, or the expiratory phase of ventilation, becomes prolonged and difficult. Special breathing tests are available to measure the amount of air that passes back and forth.

The *vital capacity* is a term used to describe how much air is brought into the lung and how much is exhaled. This capacity is markedly reduced during an asthmatic attack so that while the number of respirations per minute may be increased, the volume of air that enters and leaves the lung is reduced. It is normal for the lungs to retain a certain amount of air, called "residual air." During asthmatic attacks, this "residual" air greatly increases so there is a large collection of "stale" air in the lungs (see Figure 7).

Development of "stale" air within the lungs changes the proportion of oxygen and carbon dioxide. In protracted asthma, carbon dioxide accumulates and oxygen decreases.

Frequently recurring asthma leads to an increase in or a permanent retention of "stale" or residual air. Over a long period of time, especially if treatment has been inadequate, certain changes begin to occur in the bronchial tree.

To begin with, the smooth muscle becomes thickened and mucus plugs are more difficult to dislodge. When this occurs, the lung tissue may become scarred, decreasing the ability to inspire air.

If a large amount of residual air accumulates, the vital capacity and other breathing tests to be described later may change considerably.

Such changes, however, take many years to develop and usually are accompanied by frequently recurring infections. Most asthmatics do not progress to this stage. Asthma is different from other obstructive pulmonary diseases in that, in most asthmatics, it is reversible and an asthmatic may have long periods, even years, free from any symptoms. Andy was a good example of this. When the cause of his asthma was found to be an allergy to dust, he was treated and quickly became symptom free.

BRONCHITIS

For some, asthma is complicated by bronchitis. Although bronchitis can occur—and normally does—independently of asthma, it is often an important factor in the cause of asthmatic attacks.

The bronchitis patient may have a "rough" feeling deep inside his chest, which causes a slight stabbing pain with breathing. More often, there is a chronic cough associated with some sputum. In general, these symptoms mean there is an inflammation of the lower pulmonary passages. Fever may also occur, especially during acute attacks. Bronchitis might be pictured as continuation of a sore throat, carried downward.

The word bronchitis means inflammation of the bronchial tubes. If the trachea is involved also, the term used is tracheo-bronchitis.

Bronchitis may occur at any age and is common among infants and young children. It may be precipitated by the inhalation of irritants, including vapors, dust, and other foreign substances. "Smog" is a frequent precipitant. A severe or prolonged cold, accompanied by a cough, is the frequent sign of bronchitis. It would be accurate to say that bronchitis often has its origin after a viral infection.

EMPHYSEMA

Emphysema, considered irreversible, is a condition that begins primarily in the bronchioles and alveoli. Commonly, smokers who have chronic bronchitis develop emphysema. Smoking certainly can increase the tendency to emphysema among asthmatics, as well as non-asthmatics. When severe asthma persists over a period of years, some of the small air sacs may rupture, forming distended non-functional air sacs. If large numbers of such broken air sacs form, then residual or "stale" air increases and ventilation becomes less effective. The lung circulation also becomes altered and the vital exchange of gases may be affected. If large groups of alveoli or air sacs break down, larger air cavities may develop, with scarring of lung tissue and greatly reduced breathing efficiency.

The chest is likely to appear expanded, comparable to a position of full inspiration, and breathing becomes increasingly difficult. In time, rib cartilages tend to become rigid, the diaphragm becomes depressed, and its movement reduced. The condition is termed "barrel chest." I have heard people express the fear that they have emphysema but they don't go to a physician to see if their fears are justified. Emphysema is not a disease to leave to guesswork. If a person has emphysema, he must be treated for it, because without definite action emphysema can progress.

Emphysema may also affect the heart and circulation. The effects of emphysema on the cardiovascular system need to be evaluated for each patient. Some people with emphysema have relatively mild changes and are able to get along well, particularly when their asthma is treated and responds. This is especially important because scarring and permanent changes occur slowly, offering ample time for treatment and prevention programs.

Although *what is happening* may have a variety of causes, your primary concern is whether what is happening is mild, moderate, or severe and, in part, how long it persists. If you understand that normal ventilation is blocked during the asthmatic attack by bronchospasm, you can see how the body tries to get more oxygen by making all the chest muscles and diaphragm work harder. You need to get that oxygen to your blood cells. Retained carbon dioxide is sending messages to your brain to make you breathe harder.

Whether the process starts locally from a cellular reaction or through a reflex bronchospasm from the autonomic nerves, the degree of spasm and the amount of secretions and edema of the bronchial walls are the three important factors in how severe the attack is and how much treatment will be required.

Inflammation causing bronchitis or continuing allergic factors can add to the pathology.

Development of a meaningful program to bring your asthma

TABLE 2. Review Questions

Do I understand:
1. what asthma is?
2. why it is difficult to breathe when one has asthma?
3. what happens to the bronchial tubes in an asthmatic attack?
4. what spasm and edema are?
5. why mucus causes obstruction of air?
6. what pulmonary ventilation means?

My questions that were not answered:

---

under control requires that you become a detective. Understanding what happens to you will help in your own program.

I would like to suggest that on your worksheets you begin to list those things that you have learned from this chapter by answering the review questions in Table 2. If you find that you have listed other questions that have not been answered, place a star next to them. In subsequent chapters we shall consider the causes of asthma. If your questions are still not answered, be sure to ask your physician about them. In this manner you can complete your first goal of gaining knowledge about asthma.

3

What Causes Asthma?

"What causes asthma?" That's the question that I, as a physician, am most frequently asked.

By this time, you realize there is no single cause, but many causes. There may be a single cause in an individual asthmatic, but a variety of factors can trigger an attack. Asthma may run in families, but sometimes only one in a generation.

Determining the cause of asthma is almost always difficult, and a person's medical and emotional history may prove misleading. Multiple factors may suggest a variety of different elements as the cause, with possibly none of these the true agent. Stewart F. is an example. Stewart claimed that his first attack occurred spontaneously, without prior indication and no identifiable causative factors. Stewart is an American of English descent now living in New York, who prided himself on his strength during his twenties when he worked in a cement plant in Texas. He had his first attack six years ago while swimming off Galveston one morning after a hearty evening of drinking and dancing the night before.

"I was swimming to settle my nerves and clear my head," Stewart told me. "Then I thought, 'I've been swimming too long. I'll go back to shore.' I started to reverse myself and suddenly I had no breath—no breath at all. I thought, 'What is happening to me? I'm not going to make it. I'm going to die out here in the ocean.' Then I thought, 'I'm too young to die!' I stopped trying to swim, rolled over on my back and floated, and tried not to be frightened because it was so difficult to breathe. After a few minutes, I realized no one would ever know what happened to me because no one knew I'd gone swimming. Gradually my breathing became easier and, finally, I was able to swim back, swimming like an old man, slowly. When I came ashore, my young nephew saw me.

" 'What's wrong with you?' he demanded.

" 'I've just turned into an old man,' I said.

" 'At thirty?'

"I just nodded and collapsed in his arms. He lowered me onto the sand. It was a long time before I could walk. I weighed 165 pounds when I went swimming that morning. Today I weigh 120 pounds. Until then I could carry sacks of cement with no effort at all. Today I can hardly carry my little girl. She's only seven, born a year before I got sick. Hardly more than a baby, but I can't even pick her up. That hurts the most. I can't even pick up and carry my little girl."

Stewart's treatment for asthma is complicated by the fact that he is a heavy smoker, although he always insists he's not had a cigarette in months. Even during emergency hospital treatment for an acute attack, he has been known to sneak into the bathroom for a cigarette. He's also a heavy drinker. In consequence, his nutrition is extremely poor. Often he does not eat for a day or two at a time; he rarely eats more often than once a day. He blames his asthma for his loss of appetite, and asthma can be a factor; but, of course, it's his excessive drinking that inhibits his food intake. Stewart is intelligent and has an agreeable disposition. I've heard nurses call him "sweet"—even though they know he doesn't tell the truth when it comes to cigarettes and liquor. He has not worked in over two years and claims he would like nothing better than to be able to go back to work, yet he will not follow recommendations for treatment of asthma or alcoholism and won't give up smoking. Stewart's asthma has other psychological and physiological roots. Smoking and drinking are not the basic causes.

Lenore M. is another example of misleading features in the history.

For a long time, Lenore kept my offices in perfect dust-free order and had the great virtue of being able to tidy my desk without misplacing a paper. Then she married. Her first child was born within the year—and she worked up until the day she went to the hospital for the birth. With the baby-sitting help of a younger sister, she was back helping me within six weeks of the baby's birth. Before another year passed, a second baby was born, but this time the younger sister rebelled. Lenore had to stay home and take care of her babies herself. We parted with mutual regret.

Periodically after that she would call up and ask about certain patients who had been her favorites and about the care and well-being of some of our office plants she loved. I did not see her personally until one day when she telephoned me, gasping, "I'm sick. Very sick. I can't breathe. Please help."

Checking my bag to make sure I had adrenalin as well as other medications, I drove to Lenore's home. She opened the door. Her handsome black skin was nearly gray in color. She was in the midst of an acute asthmatic attack. But what shocked me more than that was Lenore herself. From a weight of probably 120 when she left my employ she had ballooned to a weight I estimated to be over 200 pounds.

Getting her to a chair, I quickly examined her lungs and heart and took her blood pressure. It was normal so I administered the adrenalin quickly. Within ten minutes, her breathing eased. Twenty minutes later, I gave her another injection, and shortly after that, when I listened to her lungs, all the raspings and rattles had disappeared. She no longer complained of tightness in her chest. The attack was over. Then we talked.

I asked why she had gained so much weight.

"Eating," she answered, realistically. "I am bored being at home, just with the babies, and so I eat. All day long I eat."

"Most mothers with two young babies claim they don't have time to eat," I teased her.

"They just aren't good workers," she said. "My babies are well taken care of but it isn't interesting here like it is in your office. I don't even have plants to take care of."

I asked her why she didn't buy some plants. "My husband says they cost too much," she said.

"Less than what it costs him to provide you with all that food you eat," I said.

It wasn't difficult to persuade Lenore of the wisdom of going on a diet to regain her figure—"and your health," I said. When her husband came home shortly afterward, I suggested that he and I buy her some plants for her living room and kitchen. He was ready to object but when I pointed out that her ingestion of food was costly and harmful to her health and a contributing cause of her asthmatic attack, he readily agreed.

Lenore and I have stayed in touch over the years. She never went back to work but she did lose more than seventy pounds. Was being overweight the cause of her asthmatic attack?

The implication that obesity is a cause of asthma has never been researched for most chronic asthmatics are thin. While obesity can be a cause of breathlessness, shortness of breath alone is no sign of an impending onset of asthma. If you are overweight and breathless, direct your worry toward doing something about your weight so that you'll be able to breathe easier. It might help—at least by making you smile—to tack up on your refrigerator door the oysters' plea in *Alice's Adventures in Wonderland:*

> "But wait a bit," the Oysters cried,
>   "Before we have our chat;
> For some of us are out of breath,
>   And all of us are fat."

Asthmatic symptoms are often confusing and many people who have asthma are wrong more often than not about how or when or why their asthma started, and rarely know what kind of asthma they have. In Stewart's and Lenore's cases, it certainly wasn't the swimming or weight gain that produced the asthma. Unless you delved more deeply into the stories of each, you couldn't know that Stewart had a complicated intrinsic asthma made worse by smoking and alcohol, while Lenore had an extrinsic asthma caused by allergies that increased markedly because of her weight gain.

Extrinsic and intrinsic asthma! Those are terms important to know in relation to asthma in general and your asthma in particular.

TABLE 3. Common Causes of Extrinsic Asthma

---

1. Foods, such as chocolate, fruits, nuts, milk, eggs, corn, wheat.
2. Pollens, from flowers, trees, grasses, weeds.
3. Dust, such as house and other dust.
4. Molds, from cheese, plants, soil, damp basements, etc.
5. Animal dander, from horses, cats, dogs, birds.
6. Chemicals and drugs, such as penicillin, ampicillin, aspirin.
7. Furniture, especially from kapok or goose down stuffing.
8. Cosmetics.
9. Air pollutants.

EXTRINSIC AND INTRINSIC ASTHMA

Extrinsic, which means "from the outside," refers to people who are allergic to some external material—inhalants, such as pollens and chemical fumes; ingestants, such as foods and additives; and contact allergens, such as wool, plastics, and feathers. Table 3 lists common causes of extrinsic asthma.

Intrinsic refers to asthma triggered by some internal cause, such as infection. Intrinsic asthma has been called infectious asthma because, frequently, colds or upper respiratory infections often occur before the attacks. Such individuals require repeated use of antibiotics and may have a history of sinus infections. Such asthma episodes don't occur during particular seasons, as is often the case with ex-

TABLE 4. Characteristics of Intrinsic Asthma

---

1. Frequent upper respiratory infections.
2. Repeated need for anti-spasmodic drugs.
3. Non-seasonal attacks.
4. Less frequent attacks during nice weather.
5. Increased attacks during inclement weather.
6. Negative skin tests for allergy.
7. History of tonsillitis, sinus infections, ear inflammation.
8. No response to avoidance of suspected foods or pollens.

---

trinsic asthma, but often they are aggravated during the fall and winter and disappear during the good weather of summer.

With intrinsic asthma, there is often a delay between the cause and development of the asthmatic attack, as in the case of Jessica P. Table 4 summarizes the characteristics of intrinsic asthma.

A third classification is the "mixed type," where the asthmatic has both allergies *and* infections. This is often the most difficult to manage.

Before suggesting some of the ways to describe *your* asthma, it might be well to identify some of the words used in defining allergies, their causes, and controls, since many sound alike and could be confusing:

> *Allergen*—a substance that induces allergy.
>
> *Allergy*—pathological reaction to certain foods, drugs, inhalants, and a wide variety of substances that come in contact with the skin. Parasites and viruses also can cause allergic reactions.
>
> *Antigen*—a substance that when introduced into the body stimulates production of an antibody.
>
> *Antibody*—a substance formed in the body to neutralize the antigen.

In most persons, the antigen/antibody reaction takes place without any awareness of the individual. In the allergic person, however, the antigen/antibody reaction induces a combination of chemicals that results in specific symptoms, such as asthma attacks.

It takes awhile for the body to form an antibody. Until that antibody is formed, the antigen will usually not produce allergic reactions. Sometimes sensitivity to a particular antigen is delayed months or even years. This is why a person can use a product for long periods of time with no ill effect and suddenly have an allergic reaction to it. Cosmetics are a good example. A woman can use a particular hair dye for years, and then, one day when she uses it, she can find herself sneezing or wheezing or developing a rash or another manifestation of allergy.

We don't understand what the delaying factors are or what suddenly causes a reaction when there has been no prior evidence of sensitivity to a substance. For instance, no one is allergic to penicillin on the first injection. However, sometime after that first injection or even many injections, a reaction can take place. You may be ingesting penicillin without knowing it if you drink milk from cows to which penicillin has been administered. Then, the first time you are given a penicillin injection, you may have a mild to severe reaction. You might protest to the doctor that you have never been given penicillin before; but actually the injection was not your first exposure since you had been ingesting it unknowingly.

When extrinsic asthma is the cause or a factor, usually there will be a positive reaction to skin tests. That is, when an allergist does a skin test for allergic reactions by injecting an antigen underneath the skin, he is really testing to see whether or not you have an antibody which will react with that antigen. If you do, the skin around the injection site will produce a red welt or wheal. Skin tests, however, are not infallible. You may have extrinsic causes, yet the adverse antigen/antibody factor may not be revealed by the injection of the antigen.

Michael is a case in point of a delayed antigen/antibody reaction.

Ellen K., a patient of mine, has a young son, Michael, who is the patient of a pediatrician with whom I work closely. Mrs. K and Michael were invited to the Jersey shore not long after the boy had completed a series of skin tests indicating that he was allergic to milk, chocolate, strawberries, dust, and a variety of pollens. Ellen asked about the wisdom of accepting the invitation. I suggested that they go and supported Michael's pediatrician in urging that she try not to restrict Michael's diet while on their visit.

The first week of their vacation brought a happy phone call from Ellen. Michael had not had one asthmatic attack. The second week brought a different kind of call. She and Michael were back in New York City. He had suffered such a severe asthma attack she was afraid to be away from the pediatrician. The pediatrician and I interviewed her together.

"What was different about the second week?" the pediatrician asked Ellen.

"Nothing really," said Ellen, "except that Michael's best friend, Bobby, joined us."

"Was there any trouble between them?"

"Oh, no. They are best friends."

"Because we did not restrict Michael's diet, did he eat a lot of the foods he's allergic to?" I inquired.

"No. He was very careful."

"Something was different," I said. "Did the weather change drastically? Was he exposed to a lot of dust or anything like that?"

"No, nothing like that. But yes, now that I think of it, there was something different. When Bobby joined us, he brought his pet parakeet with him. But Michael's not sensitive to birds. You remember, he had a negative reaction when he was tested to see if he was allergic to feathers. That's why we allowed Michael to give Bobby the bird for his birthday. Bobby had told Michael he wanted one and we thought it a safe gift since Michael wasn't bothered by feathers."

"Maybe Michael tested negative because, up to then, he had not had a sufficient exposure to feathers to produce an adverse reaction," I suggested. "Does he use a feather pillow?"

"No. We've never used feather pillows or anything with feathers because my husband is allergic to feathers."

"That's probably it, then," the pediatrician said. "How long has Bobby had the parakeet?"

"A few weeks. His birthday was about a month after Michael had his allergy tests."

Subsequently, Michael was tested again for feathers and for a few other items we had come to suspect since his original skin tests. Feathers proved to be the culprit. When Michael had first been tested for feathers, he had not been exposed to them so he did not demonstrate a sensitivity.

TRIGGERS

Causes of asthma, and allergy, can be easily confused with the triggers that cause the manifestations. Some people have asthmatic attacks when the air becomes humid or when it rains or when the wind blows or when the air turns cold or is heavily polluted. These are conditions that trigger attacks in some people.

Triggers, we doctors believe, probably account for a large number of episodes of so-called "unexplained asthma," which occur in the allergic person from time to time. These vary from environmental conditions to fatigue, to tension, to unreleased anger, to odors.

The trigger factor can be reduced to a formula that points up its importance in the life of an asthmatic. The severity of the attack is equal to the potency of the trigger factor *times* the intensity of the exposure *divided by* the personal resistance.

You might liken the relationship—the difference—between trigger and cause to a gun. The cause is the bullet, while the adverse situation can pull the trigger, thus producing the asthmatic attack in a sensitive person (see Figure 8).

Asking an asthmatic child to consider possible trigger factors of his attack, I said an attack can be triggered by such different things as having a cold or becoming angry.

"When we feel angry or unhappy, it can affect our entire body," I told him.

"But when I can't breathe, it makes me unhappy," the youngster responded. "Sometimes I cry."

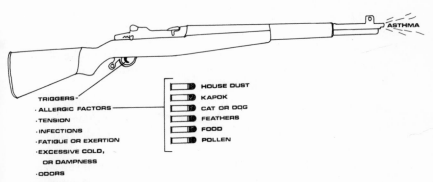

TRIGGERS IN ASTHMA

TRIGGERS·
·ALLERGIC FACTORS
·TENSION
·INFECTIONS
·FATIGUE OR EXERTION
·EXCESSIVE COLD,
  OR DAMPNESS
·ODORS

HOUSE DUST
KAPOK
CAT OR DOG
FEATHERS
FOOD
POLLEN

ASTHMA

FIGURE 8.
Trigger factors are related to causes. Without the underlying sensitivity, however, they would not initiate an asthmatic attack. To make the rifle fire, you must have a bullet *and* pull the trigger. Not shown here is that in certain people an infection may also act as a bullet.

I nodded sympathetically. "But were you unhappy, or angry, before you had the problem about breathing?"

"Sometimes," he conceded.

"If emotion can trigger an asthma attack," I said, "it's like the question that people have wondered about forever: Which comes first: the chicken or the egg?"

"The egg," the boy responded quickly.

"But who laid it?" I teased.

Emotions are a factor in most acute and lingering asthma attacks, but probably do not play a primary role. Amateur psychologists often say that all asthma is emotional in origin. That is an exaggeration unsupported by fact. But, in a number of instances, emotions may play a secondary role, particularly as trigger factors. Certain research studies do, in fact, indicate that emotions are important factors in twenty-five percent of asthmatics. Yet asthmatics have a right to be annoyed when, in the midst of an attack, friends and relations blame the attack on their "emotions," or call the attack "psychosomatic," when the asthmatic is certain that physiological conditions are involved.

A new asthmatic patient of mine, Jane J., told me that she was suffering so consistently from asthma one February that a friend of hers, a famous specialist in psychosomatic medicine, told her that she had two choices: Go to a psychiatrist for treatment or take a trip to get away from business tensions and a former husband who was constantly trying to see her. She went to Tucson, Arizona, a place she had never been before, but a city that has attracted asthmatics from all over because of its climate. Unfortunately, she arrived in the middle of a severe dust storm. Soon after checking into a hotel, she found herself in the midst of a full-blown asthma attack. Thinking she might still be suffering from the "tension" she had left behind and "bad weather," she waited until morning to consult a doctor. As she became worse, the hotel recommended that she go to the emergency room of the local hospital. She was treated and sent away, the attack broken. But that night, even though the dust storm had subsided, the attack was back as severe as ever. She returned for emergency services, but after several hours the doctors said they would have to hospitalize her for treatment.

In the hospital she improved rapidly, becoming convinced as each day brought sunshine and clear weather that her asthmatic attacks were the result of tension and unhappiness. She returned to New York prepared for intensive, long-term psychoanalysis. A variety of events delayed her therapy, and by accident she came to see me some months later.

On reviewing her story, it was apparent that Ms. J. had a long history of allergies, dating back to her late teens, and, in addition, a history of many respiratory infections. She had had a number of sinus attacks and knew that she was allergic to a number of foods. In the past she had always told her physicians (she used many, rarely returning to the same doctor more than once or twice) that she was an asthmatic and had expected that they would give her medication which would cure her rapidly.

After discussing the complexities of asthma with Ms. J., she was tested for allergies and was found to be allergic to dust, mold, and yeast. With a long history also of sinus and upper respiratory infections, she was a prime example of "mixed type" asthma, having both extrinsic and intrinsic components with tension and anxiety factors acting as triggers.

The trip to Arizona misled her into believing that her emotions were the basic cause of her asthmatic attacks. It was not until later that she began to properly sort out the different factors which can cause asthma. At that point she was able to understand how to avoid the triggers which could produce an asthmatic attack.

The "mixed" asthmatic is more difficult to treat than the person who is just allergic or who has only an infectious cause. The person with "mixed asthma" must not only learn what he is allergic to but must also try to reduce the incidence of infections, because just avoiding allergens may not be enough.

Understanding all of these factors is the first step to unravelling the details of the causes of your asthma. In Chapter 4 allergies are discussed in detail and additional examples of the role of emotions are given.

4

Allergies and Emotions

Allergies, a word coined in 1906, have been known since the beginning of recorded history. The ancient Chinese knew about allergies and asthma and wrote about their treatment. An early fatality from an allergy was King Menes of Egypt, who died in 2641 B.C., from a bee sting.

Allergies are not implicated in all asthma and many who have allergies do not have asthma. But a great many who develop asthma as adults, even late in life, often have had a long allergic history prior to the onslaught of asthma.

The Allergy Foundation of America estimates there are 35,000,000 sufferers from allergies in the United States—and they are on the increase. The loss to our national economy is estimated at many millions of man-days annually. But allergies can be identified and, when identified, they can be treated and controlled.

You do not inherit a specific allergy; rather you may belong to a family with a predisposition to become allergic. If both parents are allergic, or members of each of their families have allergies, there is greater likelihood that all or some of the children will have allergies.

However, the allergies are not necessarily the same kind as the parents' and the children's allergies may differ one from the other.

Allergy attacks may be mild, acute, or even cause death—as in the case of King Menes—if adequate medical help is not available. The attack may manifest itself in a mild case of sneezes or a skin rash that may last a few minutes, hours, days, or weeks, or in severe asthma and even complete collapse. Itches, hives, and gastrointestinal reactions are some of the common symptoms occurring in allergic persons. Many allergic persons have more than one symptom, but often breathing difficulty is the only evidence of an allergy.

ALLERGENS

Common inhaled allergens include pollens from weeds, grasses, trees, and plants; dust in the home and industry, including coal and wood dust; feathers, cosmetics, hair lotions, insecticide sprays, kapok, tobacco, many chemicals, and skin or hair shed by domestic or wild animals, including horses, cats, dogs, pigeons, and rabbits. It is important to remember that when an allergen enters the body it becomes an antigen and may produce an antibody to react with it.

Hay Fever. Some asthmatics trace their problems back to a "simple case of hay fever." Those who suffer seasonal hay fever aren't too likely to call it simple, plagued as they may be by attacks of sneezing and nasal congestion; redness, itching, swelling of the eyes; itching of the ears, mouth, nose, and throat; shortness of breath and wheezing; ringing in the ears and even loss of hearing, a condition that clears up when the "hay fever" ends.

Hay fever is a misnomer since an allergy to hay is rarely the cause and there is no fever. Generally the term hay fever refers to those allergies caused by inhalants such as plant pollens and mold spores.

Seasonal hay fever occurs chiefly in the spring, summer, and fall. Some victims have attacks during one season only, some through all four. East of the Rocky Mountains, hay fever reaches its peak between mid-August and mid-September when the ragweed plant comes into flower. Along the California-Oregon-Washington coast, hay fever from the pollens of trees, weeds, and grasses lasts almost ten months of the year.

Mold allergy is a common cause of hay fever in the Midwest due to the abundant growth of molds on wheat, oats, corn, and barley and on stored straw and hay. Attacks often occur after the harvest and extend through the winter since molds are not affected by low temperatures. Those who suffer from hay fever caused by pollens are freed from the problem when frost kills the leaves and weeds.

The severity of the hay fever attack depends upon the amount of pollen in the air and the person's degree of sensitivity. Few if any symptoms exist for the average sufferer when the day is cool, cloudy, windless, or rainy. When the weather is hot, dry, sunny, and windy, raising invisible clouds of pollens or molds, the hay fever victim is particularly miserable.

Ingestants. Among foods that commonly cause allergic reactions are lobster, crab, shrimp, chocolate, nuts, eggs, milk, corn, wheat, and even some fruits and vegetables, but these are probably rare causes of asthma, especially in adults. What may be more significant are food additives or chemical dyes.

There has been a dramatic increase in allergic reactions to drugs. Nurses and doctors generally ask, when reviewing a person's history, whether he or she is allergic to medications and, if so, to which. Usually specific inquiry is made about penicillin, that powerful wonder drug born of a mold and used in the treatment of a variety of different infections. Thousands of serious reactions to penicillin and penicillin derivatives are recorded, some of them fatal. Moreover, drugs given by injection, such as other antibiotics, serums, hormones, liver extract, and insulin products, are as likely to have a reaction when a sensitivity exists as those taken by mouth, such as laxatives, sedatives, and tranquilizers. Although many drug allergies are not associated with wheezing, a common drug such as aspirin has been implicated in asthma.

Contact Allergens. Many people are finding themselves allergic to man-made fibers in shirts, blouses, suits, and even sheets. Consequently there is revived interest in clothing made of natural silk, cotton, and wool, although many people are allergic to wool. One can regret the loss of the convenience represented by a drip-dry suit or shirt or a lovely wool skirt, but any such regret is short-lived when the cost can be a skin rash or, even more uncomfortably, a severe case of asthma.

Substances known to produce allergy when they come in contact with the skin include wool, leather, plastics, metals, rubber, dyes, resins, insecticides, and the foliage of certain weeds and plants, such as poison oak or ivy.

Internal Bacteria. The most challenging areas of sensitivity are those to bacteria harbored in the body, especially in the tonsils, throat, bronchi, and the sinuses. "Bacterial allergy" can be the trigger or even the cause of asthma attacks. It is the chief factor in intrinsic asthma.

IDENTIFYING ALLERGENS

When asthma is provoked by a single allergen, it often is possible to eliminate the agent and prevent asthma attacks indefinitely. When there are multiple causes, it is not as easy to avoid them. In many cases, it is possible, however, to desensitize a person to particular inhalants.

When food allergy is suspected, one approach to identify the cause is to eliminate many foods from the diet and after a few weeks restore them slowly, one at a time. If allergic symptoms appear when a particular food has been restored, it is common sense to omit this food from the diet entirely. Sometimes, however, after an extended period of abstinence, it is possible to reintroduce an earlier offender without reproducing allergic manifestations.

Elimination of error in identifying allergens can be a very challenging affair for anyone—trained allergist or earnest asthmatic alike. I placed an adult asthmatic with known food allergies on a stringent elimination diet. One of the foods eliminated was milk. The man's asthma disappeared. A little over two weeks later he telephoned to say he had decided to restore milk to his diet and that he had "not been bothered by asthma at all." I thought this to be a very short elimination period for there to be no asthmatic manifestations if milk actually was a cause. I asked if the milk he was now purchasing was the same as previously used.

"Absolutely," he said. "Same brand. Same carton."

"Was anything else different?" I inquired.

"I shopped at a different store," he said.

"That shouldn't matter," I said. "Did you buy anything regularly at the old store that you did not buy at the new?"

"Well, yes," he said. "The old store carried excellent cheeses. I used to buy Cheddar, Swiss, and Roquefort cheese there. I just buy Cheddar and Swiss at the new. They don't carry Roquefort. Could I have been allergic to cheese?"

"Hold on a minute," I said. "I want to check something."

I got out his chart and studied the results of his allergy tests.

"It may be that you are allergic to the Roquefort cheese," I said. "It seems apparent that you can eat cheese made from cow's milk, but Roquefort is made from sheep's milk and contains a mold. It's not likely you are allergic to sheep's milk, but you'll recall that you showed an allergic reaction to molds. Do you want to try eating a sample of the blue part of the cheese and see if you get an attack?"

"No," he said. "I'll just assume that I'm allergic to the more expensive Roquefort and don't have problems with less expensive cheeses. I don't think I'll risk the test, thank you."

Asthmatics often have wrong notions about what they're allergic to, particularly if they have not had skin tests. A lovely young woman came to me for a general checkup. In the course of taking her history, I learned she was the victim of asthmatic attacks. I persuaded her to take skin tests to see if she was allergic to anything. The tests showed her to be allergic to a number of inhalants and several foods. One of these was chocolate.

When I told her she was allergic to chocolate, she started to laugh, quietly at first and then almost hysterically. I was about to become alarmed, as tears started to roll down her cheeks. I handed her a glass of water. She drank some, wiped her eyes, and explained.

She had been dating two men regularly—one a fat, successful

businessman; the other, a thin, equally successful lawyer. Both wanted to marry her. She was totally enamored with the lawyer. However, regularly, after she had been with him, she had an asthmatic attack. She came to the conclusion that an emotional reaction was causing her attack. For her health's sake, she concluded that she should settle for the fat businessman. With him, she assumed, she would have a serene life—and health.

"I know I am in love with my lawyer friend," she said, wiping her eyes. "But I thought he made me too emotional. I thought it was because I got too excited with him that I had asthma attacks. Now I know. It was chocolate."

As I appeared mystified, she explained that her fat beau periodically brought her flowers and books, but her thin lawyer friend never failed to bring her chocolates because "he knows I love them so."

"I'm a chocolate-holic," she confessed. "I never ate any chocolates while he was with me but as soon as he left, I'd open the box of chocolates and never pay any attention to how many I was eating. Then I'd go to bed and in an hour or so I'd awake with an acute asthmatic attack. Often I had to go to the emergency hospital for treatment."

"Didn't anyone ever suggest allergy tests to you before?" I asked.

"Yes," she admitted, "but I like all food. I don't have a weight problem, so I didn't see how allergies could apply in my case. I felt it was emotions."

"Now you know," I said. "Allergy is the cause of your asthma. Chocolate is an allergen. You have extrinsic asthma."

She sent me an invitation to the wedding and married the thin lawyer, of course.

A liking for food does not mean that particular food is good for us. Alcoholics like whiskey. The fact is that the foods asthmatics like best can also be the ones they are most allergic to.

Mold is frequently the cause of breathing difficulties. Spores of mold are often in the air. They may also be in the soil of house plants, although there are products that can eliminate mold and allow you to enjoy the plants. (See the Resource List in the Appendix.)

A friend who knew I was writing this book called one morning to report that a business executive friend of hers had been taken to the hospital after several days of extremely severe asthma which did not respond to treatment.

"He's not had an asthma attack in years," she said. "He and his wife are baffled."

"What's different in their life or their home?" I asked.

"They've had a new roof put on their house," she replied, "but how could that be a factor?"

"It will probably develop that he's allergic to mold," I said. "Taking off the old roof could have caused a lot of mold to be dispersed into the atmosphere of the house."

The executive was hospitalized for several weeks. The principal offending factor did prove to be mold. He also was shown to be allergic to feathers.

Besides the new roof, the couple had also had the overstuffed furniture in their den reupholstered with goose down stuffing and they had bought a new eiderdown quilt. The combination of the mold from the roof and the increase in the use of feathers combined to induce his asthma.

THE ROLE OF EMOTIONS

It has become so popular to attribute asthma to emotional factors that many asthmatics have come to blame their nerves. The young woman who almost married the fat businessman with whom she was "calm" rather than the thin lawyer who excited her is a good example.

A brilliant young man, who finally managed to flee the home of an overprotective mother, is another example. While he had his own apartment, he noted that on those occasions when he visited her, an asthmatic attack inevitably occurred. One night after a particularly severe attack that required my seeing him, he announced he would never visit his mother again.

"I'm convinced," he said, "that my memories of her overprotectiveness are the cause of my attacks."

"Wait a minute," I said. "You never had attacks as a child. Isn't it only recently that you started having them? How many attacks have you had and when did they begin?"

"I've had four or five attacks," he answered. "They started about five months ago."

"What happened in your life at that time?" I asked.

"I got my own apartment," he said, "and my mother found herself a smaller one."

"And the attacks occur only after you are with her in her new apartment?"

"Yes."

"What's different about her new apartment?"

"Well," he said, "she did get some new furniture and she has a lot more plants than she had before. In fact, she has a tiny conservatory with special tropical plants."

We discussed his mother's newly expanded hobby and our discussion soon revealed that many of her tropical plants required misting and other types of special preparations. Then we ascertained that his asthmatic attacks began to occur within an hour to ninety minutes after he arrived at the apartment. He attributed the early tightness in his chest to a beginning emotional reaction. Generally he left her apartment to return to his own with a full-blown asthma attack, and on the two occasions he stayed overnight he had particularly severe attacks.

At my suggestion, he had skin tests and found he was not allergic to plants but that he was allergic to some spores and molds. It became apparent that the moisture in the house required by the plants attracted products to which he was allergic. His emotions had nothing to do with his asthma attacks.

When he told his mother about the likely cause of the attacks, she was first disbelieving and then angry. Priding herself on her meticulousness as a housekeeper, she felt nothing in her home could cause her son's problems.

Freed from fear that he was so immature that a visit to his mother could inspire asthma upsets, the son gave her a choice: Eliminate some of the tropical plants or forego his visits. She got rid of the suspected offenders.

"Now," the son told me a bit sheepishly, "I find myself calling Mother occasionally and inviting myself to dinner. I even take her out to dinner and we are finding that we have innumerable things to talk about. I have come to realize that I love her. More, I even like her. And I've not had a single asthma attack since."

Emotions, however, can be a very real factor in asthma. Some researchers believe that repressed hostility and anger can cause asthma attacks. Inability to "fight back" can be a factor. Frustration over inability to communicate with spouse or parent or boss can lead to an asthma attack.

A study done recently with forty asthmatic children at a summer camp helps clarify the role of emotions in asthma. At camp, the children were studied in relation to the extent of their asthma, their family environment, and their psychological background. Each asthmatic attack and the treatments were carefully recorded. At the camp, it was noted that the extent of the asthma related significantly to the degree to which aggressive behavior was expressed. Those children who required the most treatment were significantly less aggressive than those who were not timid and manifested anger.

A major factor in some of the most aggressive children was a separation from parents who would not tolerate a child's angry behavior at home and who often punished their child excessively. One child reported that she was frequently beaten with a clothesline by her mother for wrongdoings. At camp, during the entire summer, she had only one mild attack of asthma. Another child frequently had temper tantrums at camp, but no asthma attacks. Investigation showed that when he had a temper tantrum at home, his mother beat him. At camp, his tantrums were ignored. Result: no asthma, and fewer temper tantrums.

Expression, research indicates, is better than repression when it comes to reducing asthma.

We don't know precisely how emotions are involved in asthma. No one has this answer, but there is no question but that a number of psychological factors may induce an asthmatic attack. Repression of anger may produce a reaction that tips the seesaw (Figure 4, page 20) toward production of chemicals that may lead to an emotional state that induces an asthmatic attack. The *allergic* attack probably occurs because of an antigen/antibody reaction within the cell. The *emotional* attack probably has something to do with the automatic, or autonomic, nervous system, causing excessive spasm of the bronchial tubes without the cellular response. When a child (or an adult) knows he can express anger without undue punishment, he will let the anger come out and his autonomic nervous system may not have to react.

A shy, gentle, female asthmatic patient of mine worked for a brilliant man, who is very rich, very successful, and considered a "wonderful man" by his peers. He is a well-known philanthropist and a great patron of the arts. My patient, however, found that although he would unfailingly voice brief praise for certain of her accomplishments, he had little notion of the time involved for a particular piece of work. When she was hired, the man told her he expected her to make some mistakes but that she would quickly learn how to avoid them. She thought his attitude "quite wonderful." She learned, however, that his verbalized tolerance was not matched by the facts. If she made a mistake, he regularly reminded her of it, over a period of weeks. Even if she were only indirectly responsible or might not have been responsible at all, he would express his anger over the error—and complain about how much it was costing his company in time and money. She knew that the mistake was almost inevitably his fault, because while he verbalized freely, he was rarely specific. As his well-paid employee, she did not feel free to stop short his tirades and point out his role in any errors. Once we had brought out these facts, I suggested that, for her health's sake, she decide between developing the boldness to point out the error of his ways or quit her job.

After a few really serious asthma attacks, she quit. She took a job that paid her less initially, but her bills for asthma drugs stopped promptly, and she had no more costly trips to the hospital. Since quitting her job, she has been free of asthma. Her job switch came eighteen months ago. I've seen her twice since—for routine check-ups. She is healthy and ebullient, loves her new job, and has had two raises, so that now she is making more money than when working for the "wonderful" philanthropist.

Another patient of mine, from a "nice" home, where it was not considered proper to lose one's temper, had been suffering from allergy for several years when she came to me. Taking her history, I soon learned she had "mixed" asthma, being allergic to a number of inhalants and ingestants, but also having a long history of colds and sinus infections.

Her mother also had been asthmatic. The mother's story is interesting. Her asthma started from age seven, shortly after *her* mother (my patient's grandmother) died and her greatly admired father married his widowed cousin. She suffered gravely from asthma until, at age 40, she left her native state and her parents, moving with her husband and their two children more than a thousand miles away. She never again had an attack of asthma. She attributed the change in her condition to the move from a severe to a warm climate. Her husband believed the elimination of her asthma was due to the fact that she was no longer seeing her beloved father with his adored second wife. Both were wrong. The allergic components of asthma were not recognized at that time.

My patient's asthma did not develop until she left her sheltered home environment to work in New York City. Tests showed she was allergic to a number of chemicals and was particularly susceptible to attack when the weather turned cold in the city; yet, previously, as a teen-ager, she had skied and had "loved" cold weather. As we worked together to identify causes and triggers, it became clear to both of us that she was frustrated and unhappy in her job; that she found the highly charged, competitive atmosphere disturbing; that she was deeply bothered by frequent displays of temper and/or temperament by the explosive president of the sportswear firm where she was employed as executive secretary.

With my encouragement, she applied for a job as librarian—for which her college training qualified her—in a small town in Idaho. She got the job nearly three years ago, married shortly afterward, and, she wrote me recently, rarely has had another asthma attack since leaving New York City and her allergens behind. She's back to skiing and loving the cold weather. She married a man with an easy disposition. They have "never had a cross word," she writes, but, she added in her recent letter, which also reported the impending birth of a baby, "whether boy or girl, my husband and I agree the baby will be taught that it is much healthier to express hostility and dissipate it then repress it to the detriment of your physical and mental health."

My pediatrics associate was treating a young boy, who always seemed to be wheezing or about to develop an asthmatic attack. The boy's problem points up how interrelated emotions and allergies can be. He had gone through the desensitization process for his allergies—and he had many—without too much benefit. Then his mother took him to Denver. A few years later, a relative of the mother became my patient. I inquired about the boy. Was he still suffering from asthma? "No," I was told, and then I heard the story:

When the child was four, his parents were divorced. The boy remained with his mother. He had a few mild asthmatic attacks. The mother began to date and finally married another man. Now the boy's asthma attacks became severe. The child's natural father was a policeman. So was the second husband. About the time the Denver trip was planned, the second husband was injured severely in a motorcycle accident. When it was known that he would live but would be hospitalized a long time, he insisted his wife go with the boy to Denver, as they had planned. While he was hospitalized, the second husband was visited regularly by a priest who persuaded him that this marriage was sinful because his wife had been divorced. After his injuries healed and he left the hospital, he divorced his wife because they were "living in sin." Some months later the boy's mother remarried her first husband. From that day, the child never had another asthmatic attack.

I suspect that if the boy's parents had not been divorced, he would have been a child with mild allergic asthma and that he would have outgrown it without ever developing a severe attack.

Asthma is complicated. Various environmental and psychological factors can be implicated. There are a whole set of antigen/antibody reactions which probably occur through some inherited trait. In the allergic person, these reactions cause sensitivities to a variety of different substances. Often we need to become a detective to trace out all the possibilities and to interrelate them. By understanding each of these causes and how asthma produces various symptoms, you will be able to identify asthma-causing factors in your own life situation.

Before turning to Section II, I would like you to create your own CHECK LIST on a worksheet. List the questions noted on page 54 *and answer them.* Then, if you have questions about asthma that I have not covered so far, put these questions at the bottom of your check list. If the answers to your questions do not appear in Sections II and III, discuss your questions with your physician. When finished, check off the date on your asthma contract, signifying that you have completed learning about asthma in general.

CHECK LIST

General Questions:

1. What is asthma? (What is happening?) I understand:
   a) Why it is difficult to breathe during an asthma attack _____
   b) What happens in the bronchial tubes during an attack _____
   c) What edema is _____
   d) What causes mucus _____
   e) What causes the cough _____
   f) The kinds of mucus there are _____
   g) What is meant by vital capacity _____
   h) What is meant by the autonomic system _____
   i) What the sympathetic nerves are _____
   j) What the parasympathetic nerves are _____
   k) What the chemoreceptor centers are _____
   l) What pulmonary ventilation is _____

2. Why do asthma attacks occur? (Why is it happening?) I understand:
   a) Difference between "intrinsic" and "extrinsic" asthma _____
   b) Involvement of inherited factors _____
   c) What can trigger an attack _____
   d) At least five trigger factors _____
   e) The difference between asthma and emphysema _____
   f) Antigen/antibody reactions _____
   g) The relation between asthma and emotion _____
   h) How infections can also be a factor _____

3. I need answers to the following questions:

II

Understanding Your Asthma

5

Your Medical History

People who are sick sometimes remind me of *Alice in Wonderland*. They act as if they were involved in a dream and on awakening everything will be normal. Remember the Cheshire Cat in *Alice?* One of the cat's characteristics, you may recall, was its ability to appear and disappear at will, often while talking with someone. On one occasion, the cat started to fade out as Alice was talking, until the only thing left was the grin.

"Well! I've often seen a cat without a grin," thought Alice, "but a grin without a cat! It's the most curious thing I ever saw in my life!"

Asthma, it often seems to me, is an illness that is like a grin without a cat. It's such an elusive disease. Just as you decide upon a course of action, the asthma seems to disappear. Still, if it is there, you should be able to find it! But how?

Up to this point you have accumulated a lot of information about asthma in general, but you may wonder how to apply it to yourself. The answer is that, as yet, you can't. You are like the doctor who has general information but doesn't prescribe until he has pinpointed his patient's needs by taking his or her history. I urge you to do that for yourself—compile a comprehensive history about yourself.

As you write your history on your worksheets, the purpose you should keep in mind is to determine:

1. the kind of asthma you have;
2. why you have asthma;
3. why you have acute attacks;
4. what factors are involved in your attacks;
5. what principles can be employed to lessen the frequency of your attacks;
6. what your doctor can do;
7. whether allergy tests, other diagnostic tests, X-ray, etc., would be helpful for you.

Think for a moment about the four questions I suggested you ask your physician (see Chapter 1): "What happens in an asthma attack?", "Why is it happening?", "What can *we* do about what is happening?", and "What can I expect?"

We already have explored the first two questions. The third question requires exploration to diagnose the factors in your asthma. This section is devoted to helping you in your diagnosis. What your doctor can do, how you should work together with him, and whether you need special tests will be dealt with later.

What you need to know *specifically* about yourself depends upon how often you have asthmatic attacks, how severe they are, and how quickly you are able to identify and understand factors that cause the attacks.

Take your Personal Asthma Contract and under "Specific Knowledge About Myself" put three subheadings: a) My General Medical History, b) My Emotional History, and c) My Allergic History.

In this section, you will record your general medical history and explore your reactions to such factors as emotion, allergy, diet, infections, climate, and seasons. When items become recognized as potential causes for an attack, you will add them to your Personal Asthma Contract. Your asthma contract should now look like the one on the facing page.

A person's history is the most important part of a doctor's examination. Much of the information that guides the doctor comes from this history. Often the doctor can make an accurate diagnosis from the history alone, because it contains clues which, when pieced

MY PERSONAL ASTHMA CONTRACT

Name _____   Date _____

Goal I. Gain Understanding of Asthma   Date Completed

1) General Knowledge   _____

2) Specific Knowledge About Myself   _____

    a) My General Medical History

    b) My Emotional History

    c) My Allergic History

---

together and properly sorted, provide vital information about the person's external and internal environment. The addition of an emotional analysis generally completes the jigsaw puzzle, although the doctor can add, if he feels it necessary, laboratory or physical examination data in order to recommend the best possible treatment.

For you, a sufferer of asthma, it will be necessary to look at all the factors which may cause your symptoms. Remember that asthma is only a symptom of what may be a series of underlying genetic, chemical, or environmental sensitivities.

Doctors often compare certain kinds of complex conditions to an iceberg. An iceberg, you'll recall, shows only a small portion of itself above the water while the major portion lies invisible below the surface.

Asthma is like an iceberg. What you see are the symptoms, but the contributing components are likely to be the greater though invisible part. That's what makes asthma so challenging a disease.

Therefore, it is essential to know as much about you as possible in order to outline the size, character, and components of your submerged iceberg.

To help in drawing an accurate picture of yourself, your medical history will include a general review and a separate series of questions for allergy, emotions, and medications.

Under each of these headings, you must try to pinpoint elements which may play a role in your asthma and eliminate those that are not a contributing factor. Use a worksheet for each of these separate "sub-subjects." At first you will assess them independently, but later you will arrive at a composite picture. When necessary, consult with your physician to define the importance of each item in relation to your asthma.

Depending upon your background and your particular problems, you may have little or nothing to write on some of these worksheets. Some subjects may require that you use more than one worksheet. After you collect the data, you will summarize each topic on the appropriate worksheet so that you can incorporate important information into your personal asthma contract. The data will include classification of the kind of asthma you have and its causes, triggers, severity, and frequency of attacks. In your personal asthma contract, these will be identified as factors and listed as your asthma pattern. As you finish each section of your history, I will guide you in detail.

Up to this point, we have not discussed any medication or treatment that you have received. But I am certain that many of you have been seeing physicians and have had various kinds of therapy. One worksheet, therefore, must include a review of medications that you have taken, as well as a review of the different categories and kinds of drugs that are used for asthma. This general information is important because, to understand your own asthma and your options, you need to understand the general principles of drug therapy. Although the first section of this book was devoted to developing a general understanding of asthma, I feel that it is pertinent to include a discussion of general treatment in this section. Perhaps asthmatics, more than other individuals, are more aware, from bitter experience, of those agents which produce the most rapid improvement.

If an asthmatic, who has come to see me about an attack, tells me that during recent similar attacks he's been helped by a particular medication, I often give him that medication first. Anyone who has suffered from asthma any length of time at all quickly becomes familiar with pills, liquids, sprays, and various forms of injections that are used in treatment. The asthmatic often knows from his symptoms, before treatment is given, how well and how quickly he will respond to that particular medication. Usually too he knows the size of a dose he requires in order for the asthmatic attack to be broken. In Section III, we will discuss your treatment plan in detail.

To develop your general medical history, carefully read the questions that follow. Whenever your answer is "yes," write down the pertinent information on your worksheet. If your answer is "no," go immediately to the next question. For example, here is a sample question:

Do you UNDERSTAND WHAT you are TO DO? Your answer should be yes. On your worksheet, you would write: I understand what to do.

As you study the questions that follow, you will note some words are capitalized. The purpose of this is to call these words to your attention, to help you record pertinent information in your worksheet in simplified form. When you have finished, by recording the capitalized words when a question is answered in the affirmative, you should have a narrative, or story, of your background that is almost like a computer print-out for you.

Here is how a hypothetical person might begin answering questions, and compiling his medical history:

1. *Family History:*
   Have your PARENTS, GRANDPARENTS, AUNTS, UNCLES, BROTHERS, SISTERS, or CHILDREN had:
   a. (Sugar) DIABETES?
   b. CANCER, LEUKEMIA, or HODGKIN'S DISEASE?
   c. TUBERCULOSIS? (consumption or TB)
   d. HIGH BLOOD PRESSURE?
   e. HEART TROUBLE, HEART ATTACKS, or ANGINA?
   f. STROKE or APOPLEXY?

g. ALLERGY (HAY FEVER, ASTHMA, HIVES, or ECZEMA)?

h. ANEMIA, BLEEDING TROUBLE, or SICKLE CELL DISEASE?

i. CONVULSIONS, FITS, or EPILEPSY?

j. YELLOW JAUNDICE or HEPATITIS?

k. MENTAL DISEASE, RETARDATION, or NERVOUS BREAKDOWN?

The person filling out this form might have, or might have had, one or more members of his/her family with a disease in one or more of these categories. Thus, on the worksheet, he would list the category, and after that the disease, so that his worksheet might show the following:

In category b, the answer might be:

    b. Cancer.

In category e, the answer might be:

    e. Angina.

In category g, the answer might be:

    g. Hay fever, asthma, eczema.

When copied on his worksheet, this information would show:

    Family History: cancer, angina, hay fever, asthma, eczema.

You may include as much additional detail as you desire—such as the particular relative involved. Just be sure you create a clear picture for yourself. By copying the italicized headings, such as *Family History,* you will have a guide for all the categories. When you have no "yes" answers for a category, put "negative" opposite the category.

It is well to start your General Medical History form with a note about your occupation and age so that you can give it, or a copy, directly to your doctor.

Name _____Date _____

Occupation _____ Age _____

1. *Family History:*

   Have your PARENTS, GRANDPARENTS, AUNTS, UNCLES, BROTHERS, SISTERS, or CHILDREN had:

   a. (Sugar) DIABETES?
   b. CANCER, LEUKEMIA, or HODGKIN'S DISEASE?
   c. TUBERCULOSIS? (consumption or TB)
   d. HIGH BLOOD PRESSURE?
   e. HEART TROUBLE, HEART ATTACKS, or ANGINA?
   f. STROKE or APOPLEXY?
   g. ALLERGY (HAY FEVER, ASTHMA, HIVES, OR ECZEMA)?
   h. ANEMIA, BLEEDING TROUBLE, or SICKLE CELL DISEASE?
   i. CONVULSIONS, FITS, or EPILEPSY?
   j. YELLOW JAUNDICE or HEPATITIS?
   k. MENTAL DISEASE, RETARDATION, or NERVOUS BREAKDOWN?
   l. GLAUCOMA?
   m. DWARFISM or BONE DISEASE?
   n. GOUT?
   o. WORMS or PARASITES?
   p. DEAFNESS or CATARACTS before age 50?
   q. HYDROCEPHALUS (extremely large heads)?
   r. KIDNEY STONES?
   s. KIDNEY TROUBLE or BRIGHT'S DISEASE?
   t. COLOR BLINDNESS?
   u. MIGRAINE?
   v. LEAD POISONING?
   w. OTHER DISEASES that seem to run in your family?

   If there are other diseases (CYSTIC FIBROSIS, for instance, or PARKINSON'S DISEASE or MULTIPLE SCLEROSIS, etc.), list.

2. *Family History (Continued)*

   a. Are any of your BROTHERS or SISTERS DEAD?

b. Has ONE of your BLOOD RELATIVES DIED of illness (not injuries) BEFORE AGE 50?

c. MORE THAN ONE?

If more than one, list number.

d. Have NONE of your BLOOD RELATIVES DIED OF ILLNESS BEFORE AGE 50?

e. Were your PARENTS RELATED BEFORE MARRIAGE?

f. If yes, WERE they FIRST COUSINS?

g. If yes, WERE they SECOND COUSINS?

h. If neither first nor second cousins, how WERE they RELATED?

i. Are you a TWIN?

j. If yes, does your TWIN look EXACTLY LIKE you?

3. *Marital History:*

Are you:

a. MARRIED?

b. WIDOWED?

c. DIVORCED?

d. SEPARATED?

e. REMARRIED?

f. SINGLE?

HAVE you had children?

g. NONE?

h. ONE?

i. TWO?

j. THREE?

k. FOUR?

l. MORE THAN FOUR?

If any of your CHILDREN have DIED, how many:

m. ONE?

n. TWO?

o. THREE?

p. MORE THAN THREE?

If any of your children have died, state causes.

q. Do any of your CHILDREN HAVE BIRTH DEFECTS?

r. Has there been a RECENT CHANGE IN YOUR MARITAL STATUS?

s. Do you LIVE WITH your SPOUSE?

t. Or do you LIVE WITH your FAMILY?

u. Or WITH FRIENDS?

v. Or LIVE ALONE?

w. Has there been a RECENT CHANGE IN THE WAY you LIVE or WHERE you LIVE?

If yes, was this DUE TO:

x. FAMILY?

y. JOB?

z. HEALTH?

aa. OTHER?

If other, state reason.

bb. Are you a COLLEGE GRADUATE?

cc. If not, are you a HIGH SCHOOL GRADUATE?

dd. If not, DID you COMPLETE ELEMENTARY SCHOOL?

If the answer to "dd" is no, put on your worksheet: DID NOT COMPLETE ELEMENTARY SCHOOL.

4. *Birth, Environment, and Activity:*

Were you BORN:

a. IN the UNITED STATES? (include Hawaii and Alaska)

b. IN CANADA?

c. IN MEXICO?

d. IN the CARIBBEAN?

e. IN CENTRAL or SOUTH AMERICA?

f. IN EUROPE or GREAT BRITAIN?

g. IN the MIDDLE EAST?

h. IN INDIA or PAKISTAN?

i. ORIENT? or other parts of ASIA?

j. AFRICA?

k. AUSTRALIA or NEW ZEALAND?

In the place where you live, is your HEALTH AFFECTED by:

l. AIR POLLUTION?

m. MOLDS from inadequate drainage?

n. DUST or DIRT?

o. Does your HEALTH LIMIT YOUR ACTIVITY?

If yes, state how. If BECAUSE OF ASTHMA, so state or indicate other reason. If yes because of ASTHMA, DOES it LIMIT:

    p. KIND OF WORK you do?

    q. KIND OF SPORTS you participate in?

    r. Where you VISIT OR TRAVEL?

    s. Do you get REGULAR EXERCISE?

If the answer is no, write on your worksheet: DO NOT GET REGULAR EXERCISE.

5. *Work:*

Are you NOW:

a. SUPPORTING yourSELF?

Supporting yourself AND OTHERS, INCLUDING:

b. SPOUSE?

c. PARENTS or PARENT?

d. CHILD or CHILDREN?

e. OTHERS?

Are you:

f. SUPPORTED BY your SPOUSE?

g. SUPPORTED BY your PARENTS?

h. EMPLOYED or WORKING?

i. DISABLED or UNEMPLOYED?

j. RETIRED?

k. HOMEMAKER?

l. STUDENT?

If you work, how many HOURS do you WORK A WEEK?

m. OVER 60 hours?

n. 40 TO 60 hours?

o. 25 TO 39 hours?

p. LESS THAN 25 hours?

q. WOULD you LIKE TO WORK MORE HOURS than you do?

r. If yes, you are PREVENTED BY REASON OF PHYSICAL CONDITION?

s. Have you ever been REFUSED or asked to PAY HIGHER THAN NORMAL LIFE INSURANCE PREMIUMS?

If yes, state if FOR ASTHMA or other reason.

t. Are you receiving DISABILITY PAYMENTS?

If yes, state if for ASTHMA or other reason.

u. Were you ever REJECTED FOR MILITARY SERVICE?

If yes, state if for ASTHMA or other reason.

6. *Constitutional, Dietary:*

In the PAST THREE MONTHS, has your APPETITE:

a. INCREASED?

b. DECREASED?

In the PAST SIX MONTHS, have you:

c. LOST OVER TEN POUNDS?

d. GAINED OVER TEN POUNDS?

e. In the PAST YEAR, have you been following a SPECIAL DIET?

If yes, indicate reason.

f. Do you DRINK MORE THAN FOUR CUPS OF COFFEE or TEA DAILY?

g. Do you EAT TWO OR MORE MEALS every day?

h. Do you EAT BREAKFAST?

i. Do you EAT MEAT, EGGS, FISH, or POULTRY nearly every day?

j. Do you EAT FRESH (RAW) FRUIT AND VEGETABLES nearly every day?

k. Do you EAT COOKED VEGETABLES nearly every day?

l. Do you FREQUENTLY SNACK BETWEEN MEALS?

If yes, are your SNACKS USUALLY:

m. CAKES or COOKIES or PIE?

n. SOFT DRINKS?

o. CANDY?

p. FRUIT or JUICES?

q. NUTS?

r. ICE CREAM or SOFT CUSTARD?

s. FRESH FRUIT or VEGETABLE JUICES?

t. Which of these foods do you ALMOST NEVER EAT?

    1) MEAT

    2) CANDY

    3) MILK

    4) SODAS

    5) FRUIT

    6) FRUIT JUICES

    7) ALCOHOL

    8) GREEN VEGETABLES

    9) CAKES, PIES, COOKIES

    10) YELLOW VEGETABLES

    11) POTATO CHIPS, PRETZELS

    12) BREAD, CEREALS

68UNDERSTANDING YOUR ASTHMA

7. *Alcohol and Drugs:*
   a. In the past year, did you DRINK any ALCOHOL?
   If yes, was the AVERAGE DAILY NUMBER OF DRINKS:
   b. OVER 7
   c. 5 TO 7
   d. 2 TO 4
   e. ONE OR NONE
   f. Does your SPOUSE HAVE A DRINKING PROBLEM?
   g. Do you have A CHILD or CHILDREN WITH A DRUG PROBLEM?
   h. Do you have a CLOSE RELATIVE WITH A DRUG PROBLEM?

8. *Smoking:*
   a. Are you a SMOKER now, or HAVE you SMOKED WITHIN THE PAST SIX MONTHS?
   If yes, have you:
   b. RECENTLY CUT DOWN on smoking?
   c. RECENTLY STARTED SMOKING MORE?
   d. Do you SMOKE (ONLY) PIPE or CIGARS?
   e. Do you SMOKE CIGARETTES?
   If you smoke cigarettes, do you:
   f. Smoke OVER 2 PACKS DAILY?
   g. Smoke 1 TO 2 PACKS DAILY?
   h. Smoke LESS THAN 1 PACK A DAY?
   If you smoke cigarettes, have you been:
   i. Smoking OVER 10 YEARS?
   j. Smoking 5 TO 10 YEARS?
   k. Smoking LESS THAN 5 YEARS?
   l. DID you SMOKE prior to six months ago, BUT are NOT SMOKING NOW?

9. *Medications History (Non-asthmatic):*
   Which medicines HAVE you TAKEN in the past?
   a. DAILY ASPIRIN, BUFFERIN, ANACIN, TYLENOL, or such?
   b. SEDATIVE, NERVE PILLS, or TRANQUILIZERS?
   c. "PEP PILLS," DIET PILLS, STIMULANT PILLS?
   d. HAY FEVER MEDICINE, SPRAYS, SHOTS?
   e. DIABETES PILLS or INSULIN SHOTS?
   f. HIGH BLOOD PRESSURE, WATER PILLS, or SHOTS?

g. HEART MEDICINE, DIGITALIS, NITROGLYCERIN?

h. BLOOD THINNER PILLS, such as Coumadin?

i. CODEINE, MORPHINE, or other NARCOTIC?

j. THYROID DRUGS?

k. HORMONE PILLS or SHOTS?

l. Cortisone or other "STEROIDS" like Prednisone?

HAVE you TAKEN:

m. ANTIBIOTICS ("sulfa" drugs, etc.)?

n. COUGH MEDICINE?

o. IRON MEDICINE, VITAMINS, or TONICS?

p. STOMACH MEDICINES, ANTACIDS, etc.?

q. HORSE SERUM (for tetanus or lockjaw)?

r. Any OTHER medicines or shots?

If so, list.

s. HAVE you HAD REACTIONS to any of these drugs?

If so, list.

t. HAVE you ever USED MARIJUANA, LSD, SPEED, REEFERS, POT?

u. If yes, mention if regularly.

v. Have you RECEIVED RADIOISOTOPES (atomic cocktail)?

IN the PAST FIVE YEARS, HAVE you HAD:

w. SMALLPOX VACCINATION?

x. All THREE ORAL POLIO VACCINATIONS?

y. TETANUS (lockjaw) BOOSTER or series?

10. *Previous Illnesses:*

HAVE you ever HAD:

a. CANCER, TUMOR, or LEUKEMIA?

b. MALARIA or OTHER TROPICAL DISEASES (worms, etc.)?

c. GERMAN or three-day MEASLES (rubella)?

d. MONO (MONONUCLEOSIS)?

e. RHEUMATIC FEVER, ST. VITUS'S DANCE, or CHOREA?

f. SICKLE CELL ANEMIA?

g. SCARLET FEVER?

h. VENEREAL DISEASE (syphilis, gonorrhea)?

i. POLIO (poliomyelitis)?

j. TYPHOID fever?

k. HEPATITIS?

l. CHICKEN POX?

m. MUMPS?

n. SMALLPOX?

o. DYSENTERY?

p. OTHER SERIOUS ILLNESSES not already listed that required long bed rest?

If yes, please list.

q. Have you ever been HOSPITALIZED?

If yes, list number of times, year(s), and reason(s). If surgery was performed, list below under Section 11.

11. *Surgical Procedures:*

a. Have you ever HAD AN OPERATION or surgery of any kind?

If yes, indicate which operations you have had and indicate year(s) the surgery took place.

b. APPENDIX

c. TONSILS and/or ADENOIDS

d. HEAD, EYES, EAR, NOSE, SINUS, MASTOID

e. BRAIN TUMOR

f. NECK or THYROID

g. CHEST

h. Chest (HEART or LUNGS)

i. ARTERIES or VEINS

j. BONES, JOINTS, BACK, or SPINE

k. RECTUM, ANUS, HEMORRHOIDS (piles)

l. HERNIA or RUPTURE

m. KIDNEY

n. BLADDER

o. GALL STONES

p. PROSTATE GLAND

q. STOMACH

r. BOWEL

s. OTHER (specify)

Note: Female organ surgery is listed later.

12. *Head, Eyes, Nose, Throat:*

a. Have you ever been knocked UNCONSCIOUS FROM A HEAD INJURY so that you were out more than five minutes?

b. Have you RECENTLY been TROUBLED BY SEVERE HEADACHES?

c. Have you ever had BLACKOUTS (other than from excessive drinking), CONVULSIONS, FITS, SEIZURES, or EPILEPSY?

d. Do you OFTEN get so DIZZY—even for a few moments—that you or the room seems to spin around (vertigo)?

e. Have you ever HAD TROUBLE WITH YOUR EYES or VISION?

If yes, has the trouble been CORRECTED BY GLASSES or MEDICINE?

f. Have you had RECENT EYE PAIN, EYE or VISION TROUBLE?

g. Do you HAVE GLAUCOMA (increased pressure in the eyes)?

h. Do you SEE COLORED HALOS around lights?

i. Do you ever SEE DOUBLE (double vision)?

j. Are you COLOR BLIND?

k. Have you ever HAD EAR INFECTIONS from a cold?

l. Have you ever HAD AN EAR INJURY or HEARING LOSS?

If yes, specify.

m. Have you ever HAD REPEATED BUZZING (ringing) IN the EARS?

n. Have you ever HAD TROUBLE WITH your BALANCE?

o. Have you had FREQUENT SNEEZING SPELLS, or HAY FEVER, or OVER THREE COLDS A YEAR?

p. Do you FAINT FREQUENTLY?

q. Have you been TROUBLED BY NOSE BLEEDS, LOSS OF SMELL, or suffered long from STUFFY OR RUNNING NOSE?

HAVE you recently noted:

r. SORES IN MOUTH, LIPS, TONGUE?

s. LUMPS IN or UNDER the TONGUE or ON or UNDER THE LIPS?

t. SORE THROAT without a cold?

u. HOARSENESS NOT DUE TO A COLD?

v. SORE TONGUE, MOUTH, or BLEEDING GUMS?

w. Do your TEETH or DENTURES give you TROUBLE?

x. Do you have SWOLLEN GLANDS or LUMPS IN your NECK NOW?

y. Have you RECEIVED RADIATION or COBALT THERAPY TO your NECK OR UPPER CHEST?

z. Is SWALLOWING DIFFICULT OR PAINFUL?

13. *Skin:*

HAVE you HAD any of these skin troubles:

a. RASHES on the body?

    b. ABNORMAL TIGHTNESS OF THE SKIN?

    c. HARD LUMPS ON the SKIN?

    d. SKIN INFECTIONS or BOILS?

    e. CONSTANT ITCHING OF the SKIN?

    f. SORES THAT DON'T HEAL?

    g. HAVE you ever HAD A BAD REACTION TO A BEE OR WASP STING?

    h. Do you now have MOLES ON your SKIN?

    If yes, are any of your moles GROWING DARKER or GETTING LARGER?

    i. Are your FINGERNAILS RIDGED?

14. *Breasts (both men and women answer):*

    a. Do you HAVE a LUMP or TUMOR or UNUSUAL SWELLING IN YOUR BREAST?

    b. HAVE you had a DISCHARGE FROM A NIPPLE DURING the PAST YEAR?

    c. Did you PREVIOUSLY have A BREAST LUMP WHICH IS NOW GONE?

    If yes, did It:

    d. DISAPPEAR SPONTANEOUSLY?

    e. Or was it REMOVED BY SURGERY?

    f. Or was any OTHER FACTOR INVOLVED in its disappearance?

15. *Blood and Lymph Glands:*

    a. IN the LAST SIX MONTHS have you HAD A SWOLLEN LYMPH GLAND IN your ARMPIT or GROIN?

    b. HAVE you drenched your bed sheets from NIGHT SWEATS?

    c. Have you been TOLD that you HAVE TOO MANY RED OR WHITE CELLS?

    d. Have you been TOLD that you HAVE ANEMIA (low blood count)?

    e. Have you been TOLD you HAVE TOO FEW WHITE BLOOD CELLS?

    f. HAVE you ever BLED EXCESSIVELY WITH OPERATIONS?

    g. Have you ever been TOLD you are a BLEEDER or HAVE HEMOPHILIA?

16. *Lungs:*

    a. HAVE you HAD CLOSE CONTACT WITH anyone (spouse or family or lover) with TUBERCULOSIS?

    b. HAVE you ever HAD TUBERCULOSIS?

    c. HAVE you ever HAD a SKIN TEST FOR TUBERCULOSIS?

d. If yes, was it POSITIVE or NEGATIVE?

Have you ever been TOLD you HAD:

e. LUNG INFECTION?

f. PLEURISY?

g. BRONCHITIS?

h. EMPHYSEMA?

i. CHRONIC LUNG DISEASE (other than asthma)?

j. FUNGUS DISEASE OF the LUNG, such as histoplasmosis?

k. If you HAVE ASTHMA, what year was it DIAGNOSED?

In the past six months, do you GET SO SHORT OF BREATH THAT IT:

l. INTERFERES WITH your USUAL ACTIVITY?

m. OCCURS EVEN AT REST?

n. OCCURS CLIMBING STEPS?

o. HAVE TO PROP UP TO SLEEP?

p. Are you TROUBLED WITH FREQUENT COUGHING?

If yes, do you COUGH UP MUCH THICK GREEN OR YELLOW SPUTUM?

q. Do you SOMETIMES COUGH UP BLOOD?

r. Have you ever HAD A CHEST X-RAY?

If yes, have you been told that your chest X-ray was NOT NORMAL?

s. Do you SUFFER FROM MANY HEAVY CHEST COLDS?

t. Is your BREATHING USUALLY NOISY WITH WHEEZING or WHISTLING sounds?

u. Is your breathing noisy with wheezing or whistling sounds only OCCASIONALLY? Or RARELY?

When you have ASTHMATIC ATTACKS, do they OCCUR in:

v. ALL SEASONS?

w. SUMMER?

x. FALL?

y. WINTER?

z. SPRING?

aa. COLD WEATHER or COLD BREEZES or air?

bb. DUSTY SURROUNDINGS?

cc. DAMP WEATHER?

Do your ASTHMATIC ATTACKS DISAPPEAR WHEN you:

dd. TRAVEL?

If so, state where.

ee. LEAVE WORK or HOME?

If so, state if any special room.

ff. ELIMINATE COSMETICS or CERTAIN CLOTHES or CERTAIN FOODS?

17. *Heart and Circulation:*

a. IN the PAST YEAR, have you HAD REPEATED DISCOMFORT or PAIN (pressure or tightness) IN your CHEST WHEN you are NOT HAVING AN ASTHMATIC ATTACK?

If yes, have you had this discomfort:

b. WHILE SITTING STILL?

c. WHEN EXCITED OR ANGRY?

d. AFTER EATING A BIG MEAL?

e. WHEN WALKING FAST OR UPHILL?

f. AFTER PHYSICAL EXERTION?

If yes, does THE DISCOMFORT:

g. AWAKEN you FROM SLEEP?

h. FORCE you TO STOP WALKING?

i. LEAVE AFTER a FEW MINUTES REST?

j. LAST OVER 10 MINUTES?

k. Does your HEART often THUMP or RACE AT REST? (Exclude if only after asthmatic medication.)

l. Do LEG CRAMPS WAKE you AT NIGHT?

m. Does WALKING MAKE YOUR LEGS ACHE so much that you must stop, but then do you feel RELIEVED AFTER A SHORT REST?

Has a DOCTOR ever SAID you HAD:

n. HEART ATTACK (CORONARY, ANGINA, CLOT)?

o. ABNORMAL ELECTROCARDIOGRAPH (ECG or EKG)?

p. HEART MURMUR?

q. HIGH BLOOD PRESSURE (hypertension)?

r. ENLARGED HEART?

s. CONGESTIVE HEART FAILURE?

t. Do you SUFFER WITH HOT or SWEATY FLASHES? (Exclude if related to "changes" or menopause.)

u. Do you HAVE VARICOSE VEINS IN the LEGS?

v. Do both your ANKLES SWELL very much?

w. If not both, does ONE ANKLE or LEG SWELL?

x. If your FINGERS GET COLD, do they BECOME NUMB, PAINFUL, DEAD WHITE, or BLUE?

18. *Stomach (Gastro-intestinal Tract):*
    a. Do you HAVE PAIN, INDIGESTION, HEARTBURN, or CRAMPS IN YOUR AB-DOMEN (stomach or belly)?
    If yes, does this discomfort occur:
    b. ON the RIGHT SIDE?
    c. ON the LEFT SIDE?
    d. ABOVE the NAVEL (belly button)?
    e. IN the CENTER?
    f. BELOW the NAVEL?
    g. If yes, does it come on WHILE or RIGHT AFTER EATING?
    h. Or does it come on ONE TO TWO HOURS AFTER EATING?
    i. Is it MADE WORSE BY BENDING OVER OR LYING DOWN?
    j. Does it FOLLOW EATING SWEETS, PIES, or FRIED or GREASY FOODS?
    k. Does it FOLLOW MEDICATION?
    If so, specify.
    Were these PAINS, CRAMPS, HEARTBURN, or INDIGESTION HELPED or RE-LIEVED BY:
    l. MILK, FOOD, SODA, or ANTACIDS?
    m. HAVING A BOWEL MOVEMENT?
    n. Were these discomforts NOT HELPED BY MEDICINES?
    Is your STOMACH UPSET:
    o. MORE THAN ONCE A WEEK?
    p. LESS OFTEN BUT FREQUENTLY?
    q. ONLY OCCASIONALLY?
    r. Are you OFTEN NAUSEATED or SICK AT STOMACH, or do you OFTEN VOMIT?
    If yes, does the VOMIT LOOK LIKE COFFEE GROUNDS or BLOOD?
    s. HAVE you HAD JAUNDICE (yellow eyes or skin)?
    t. HAVE you FREQUENT LOOSE STOOLS (diarrhea)?
    u. HAVE your BOWEL MOVEMENTS been BLACK AS TAR even when not taking iron pills?
    v. HAVE you HAD a RECENT CHANGE IN BOWEL HABITS?
    w. Are you often AWAKENED AT NIGHT TO DEFECATE (have a bowel movement)?

x. HAVE YOU HAD MUCUS IN your BOWEL MOVEMENTS?

y. HAVE YOU HAD, or do you now HAVE, HEMORRHOIDS (piles) or RECTAL CRACKS?

z. HAVE YOU HAD PAIN, ITCHING, or BURNING of the RECTUM?

aa. HAVE YOU HAD OTHER TROUBLES WITH BOWEL MOVEMENTS?

bb. HAVE YOU HAD STOMACH or DUODENAL or PEPTIC ULCERS?

Have you been TOLD that you HAD, or HAVE:

cc. BOWEL or COLON DISEASE?

dd. HEPATITIS, CIRRHOSIS, GALL BLADDER, or OTHER LIVER DISEASE or PAN-CREATITIS?

ee. IN THE PAST FIVE YEARS, HAVE YOU HAD X-RAYS TAKEN OF your GALL BLADDER, STOMACH, or INTESTINES?

19. *Urinary Tract:*

a. Do you USUALLY HAVE TO GET UP FROM SLEEP TO URINATE (pass water)?

b. Do you URINATE EVERY FEW HOURS DURING THE DAY?

c. During the PAST YEAR, has URINATION CAUSED PAIN OR BURNING?

d. Do you OFTEN HAVE such URGENCY TO URINATE you cannot wait to get to the bathroom?

e. HAVE YOU LOST CONTROL of your BLADDER?

If yes, did you lose control WHEN:

f. You were COUGHING (in an asthma attack)?

g. You were UNABLE TO GO to the bathroom FOR MANY HOURS (for any reason)?

h. You were LAUGHING?

i. There would appear to be NO REASON?

j. Have you been TOLD that you HAVE A KIDNEY or BLADDER STONE?

k. Is your URINE STREAM WEAKENED SO THAT IT JUST DRIBBLES?

l. Does your URINE CONTAIN BLOOD, PUS, or is it VERY DARK or DIS-COLORED or does it turn BLACK?

m. Are there TIMES WHEN you felt that your bladder was full but NO URINE WOULD PASS?

20. *Genital Tract:*

a. HAVE YOU HAD AN OPERATION TO PREVENT PREGNANCY?

b. HAVE YOU HAD any TROUBLE WITH GENITALS (sex organs)?

c. HAVE YOU HAD any PHYSICAL SEX PROBLEMS of any kind?

d. HAVE YOU HAD PROSTATE GLAND TROUBLE?

21. *Nervous System:*
    a. Has your SPEECH CHANGED so you can no longer talk without slurring words?
    b. Do you LOSE YOUR ABILITY TO SPEAK for a few minutes?
    c. Do you LOSE TRACK OF HAPPENINGS around you?
    d. HAVE you HAD a PECULIAR TASTE OR SMELL for no reason?
    e. WHEN you COUGH or SNEEZE or have an asthma attack, do you GET A PAIN IN your BACK?

    If yes, is the pain in:

    f. LOWER BACK?
    g. BETWEEN THE SHOULDER BLADES?
    h. Have you found you have LOST your POWER TO enunciate (SAY) COMMON WORDS?
    i. Do you OFTEN HAVE NUMBNESS OF your FACE, HANDS, or LEGS?
    j. Are you IN CONSTANT PAIN?
    k. Have you become CLUMSY so that you find you can't button buttons?
    l. Do you HAVE TROUBLE CONTROLLING your LEGS IN WALKING?
    m. Do you HAVE a CONSTANT shaking (TREMOR) OF your HEAD or HANDS?
    n. Have you been TOLD that you HAVE HAD a STROKE (apoplexy)?
    o. Do you now HAVE UNUSUAL WEAKNESS OF ONE SIDE OF your FACE, ONE ARM, or ONE LEG?

22. *Bones and Joints:*
    a. Have you HAD RECENT PAIN IN your BACK SO you COULDN'T DO WORK?
    b. Are your JOINTS STIFF or PAINFUL WHEN you WAKE UP?
    c. Have you been TOLD that you HAVE ARTHRITIS?
    d. Have you been TOLD that you HAVE, or HAVE HAD, GOUT?
    e. Are you SO STIFF that you CAN'T BEND JOINTS OF the BACK, or STRAIGHTEN UP AS you USED TO be able to do?
    f. In the PAST YEAR, HAVE you been TROUBLED WITH A PAINFUL STIFF NECK?
    g. HAVE you ever HAD A BONE INFECTION (osteomyelitis)?
    h. HAVE you recently HAD FREQUENT PAIN IN YOUR JOINTS?
    If yes, SPECIFY which joints.
    i. In the PAST YEAR, HAVE you HAD SWOLLEN or RED JOINTS?
    If yes, SPECIFY which joints.
    j. Are your MUSCLES SWOLLEN or TENDER?

k. Are your MUSCLES WEAK or WASTED (shrunken)?

l. Do you SUFFER WITH MUSCLE CRAMPS?

m. Have you HAD a BONE OR JOINT OPERATION?

If yes, specify, if not already listed under Section 11: Surgical Procedures.

n. HAVE YOU HAD MORE THAN ONE BROKEN BONE?

If yes, list which and dates when bone(s) broken.

23. *Endocrine Glands:*

   a. Have you ever been TOLD that you HAD sugar DIABETES, SUGAR IN your URINE, or BLOOD IN your URINE?

   b. Have you ever been TOLD that you HAVE HYPOGLYCEMIA (low blood sugar)?

   c. Are you CONSTANTLY THIRSTY and always need to drink water or other liquids?

   d. SINCE you became an ADULT, and not from fat, has your HEAD, GLOVE, or SHOE SIZE INCREASED?

   e. Do you LOSE WEIGHT even THOUGH you HAVE a big APPETITE and eat a normal or even more than normal amount of food?

   f. Do you HAVE a GOITER (enlarged thyroid gland)?

   g. Have you been TOLD that you HAVE an OVERACTIVE THYROID?

   h. Have you been TOLD that you HAVE an UNDERACTIVE THYROID?

   i. Is your BODY usually MOIST or SWEATY?

   j. Is your BODY HOTTER than it used to be?

   k. Is your BODY COLDER than it used to be?

   l. In the PAST YEAR, do you HAVE a CRAVING FOR SALT even without food?

   m. HAVE YOU HAD a great CHANGE IN SKIN COLOR or TEXTURE?

   n. HAVE YOU HAD a recent INCREASE in the amount of FACIAL HAIR?

   o. HAVE YOU HAD a recent DECREASE in the amount of FACIAL HAIR?

   p. HAVE YOU LOST most of the HAIR UNDER YOUR ARMS or ABOUT THE SEX ORGANS?

24. *Questions for Women Only:*

   a. Have NEVER HAD A PERIOD.

   b. STARTED BEFORE 10 YEARS OLD.

   c. STARTED BETWEEN 10 AND 17 years of age.

d. STARTED AFTER 17.

e. Are you STILL HAVING PERIODS?

If yes, are your periods REGULAR? IRREGULAR?

f. Do you SKIP PERIODS?

g. Are your PERIODS EVERY 25 TO 30 DAYS?

h. Are your periods MORE OFTEN THAN EVERY 25 TO 30 DAYS?

i. Or is it MORE THAN 30 DAYS from the beginning of one period to the start of the next?

If you are still having PERIODS, how long do they LAST?

j. 4 TO 6 DAYS.

k. LESS THAN 4 DAYS.

l. OVER 6 DAYS.

m. Do you HAVE VERY HEAVY PERIODS, or ABNORMAL BLEEDING, so that you ever need more than ten regular pads, or tampons, for any one twenty-four-hour period?

n. Are your PERIODS ever, or sometimes, PAINFUL to the point they are bothersome?

o. Do you FEEL BLOATED OR IRRITABLE A WEEK BEFORE your PERIOD?

p. HAVE you RECENTLY STOPPED HAVING MENSTRUAL PERIODS?

q. Do you THINK you are PREGNANT NOW?

r. If you have ever been pregnant HAVE you HAD any BABY WEIGH NINE OR MORE POUNDS?

s. If you have had a baby, HAVE you BREAST FED A BABY FOR MORE THAN THREE MONTHS?

t. HAVE you HAD A URINARY INFECTION WHILE PREGNANT?

u. HAVE you HAD TOXEMIA OR ECLAMPSIA WHILE PREGNANT?

v. HAVE you HAD SUGAR IN YOUR URINE WHILE PREGNANT?

w. AFTER DELIVERY, did you GAIN WEIGHT QUICKLY?

x. HAVE you ever HAD a MISCARRIAGE?

If so, how many?

y. HAVE you ever HAD an ABORTION?

If so, how many?

z. Is "CHANGE OF LIFE" GIVING you TROUBLE?

aa. Do you get "DRAGGING DOWN" feelings IN your ABDOMEN (belly) and BACK?

bb. Within the PAST 12 MONTHS, HAVE you HAD a "PAP" OR CANCER SMEAR?

25. *Surgery:*

HAVE YOU HAD:

a. BREAST SURGERY?

b. SCRAPING OF THE WOMB (D&C)?

c. REMOVAL OF ALL OF PART OF the WOMB (uterus)?

d. OPERATION ON a TUBE OF OVARY?

e. CANCER OF the BREAST? A BENIGN TUMOR OF the BREAST?

f. SURGERY FOR CANCER OF the UTERUS (womb) or CERVIX?

g. RADIUM OF X-RAY TREATMENT OF the FEMALE ORGANS?

h. OTHER FEMALE ORGAN OF BLADDER OPERATIONS?

If so, specify.

i. OTHER TROUBLE with FEMALE ORGANS?

j. PHYSICAL DIFFICULTIES with SEX LIFE?

You have now completed a major portion of your medical history. Many of the questions listed above will seem to you far afield from the subject of asthma. But whenever you have a "yes" answer to any question, it may be important. A medical history needs to be complete. If you have other problems, they could interfere with your asthma and with the attainment and maintenance of optimum health. Actually every individual can be benefited by creating such a comprehensive medical history. As you note the detail and extent of the questions, you will see that the history you are recording is similar to a comprehensive medical history taken by a doctor. Because your goal is preventive medicine, your doctor may welcome this information if he does not already have it.

Look over your history. You may find that in each category there are occasional responses which do not seem to add up to any kind of pertinent story. This is not uncommon. It is not significant.

What *is* important is whether you can identify common *recurring* features in your history, which may be associated with asthmatic attacks. This is especially true of the social, environmental, and family backgrounds of many patients. If you can identify any such recurring features, *star* or *circle* them on your worksheets because later you may transfer all or some of them to your personal asthma contract. For example, see the items marked by a star * on the John Jones sample history on page 82.

Finally, it is possible that taking your history may make you aware of a number of complaints in one or two or more of the categories, such as heart and circulation, or endocrine glands. If so, it is imperative that you check these with your physician to be certain that a new problem does not exist that could be important to your well-being and which may or may not be an underlying factor in your asthma.

Especially important in relation to asthma are those questions which suggest recurring infection. Frequent headaches, particularly in central parts of the head, might suggest a recurring sinus condition. Be especially on guard for this possibility if it seems that, when you have a headache, your upper teeth also seem to hurt. Maxillary sinus infection often feels like a toothache over a cheek.

Frequent colds, sore throats, enlarged glands, recurring fever, and sputum which has a yellowish or greenish tinge may be additional signs of infection. Later, when you review medications that you have taken, strongly suspect an infection if your doctor frequently prescribes antibiotics, such as penicillin or the mycins. The John Jones sample worksheet that follows is an example of the kind of information that suggests recurring infection.

You will note that the worksheet contains every one of the major headings from the General Medical History Form. When no problem exists in any one category, the word "negative" appears opposite it. When the respondent is a male, as in the case of the John Jones sample history, the words "not applicable" appear opposite the category that is for women only.

(SAMPLE)

GENERAL MEDICAL HISTORY

Name: John Jones   Date: Jan. 10, 19—
Age: 21   Occupation: Student

Family History: Mother has high blood pressure.
Marital History: Single.
Birth, Environment, and Activity: Born U.S.
                                  Health affected by pollution in air, dust.

Do not get regular exercise.

Have limitation of work, sports, because of asthma.

Work: Supported by parents.

Dietary: Drink more than four cups of coffee daily.

Eat three meals a day.

Eat meat, poultry, fish, or eggs every day.

Eat cooked and/or raw vegetables nearly every day.

Eat raw fruit several times a week.

Like doughnuts, cake, cookies.

Rarely eat candy, potato chips.

Rarely drink soft drinks or hard liquor.

Alcohol and Drugs: Sometimes drink wine.

Smoking: Don't smoke.

Medications History: *Have taken antibiotics and cough medicine frequently.

Previous Illnesses: Have had:

Mononucleosis.

German measles.

Chicken pox.

Hospitalized once—mono.

Surgical Procedures: *Had tonsils removed.

Head, Eyes, Nose, Throat: *Had ear infection.

*Had recent sore throat.

*Have had swollen glands in neck often.

Skin: Negative.

Breasts: Negative.

Blood and Lymph Glands: Negative.

Lungs: Asthma diagnosed in 1970. Short of breath with wheezing, whistling sounds.

Heart and Circulation: Negative.

Stomach:	Negative.
Urinary Tract:	Negative.
Genital Tract:	Negative.
Nervous System:	Negative.
Bones and Joints:	Negative.
Endocrine Glands:	Negative.
Questions for Women Only:	Not applicable.

I have mentioned your doctor several times. I think it is important for me to stress again how I feel you and your physician should work together.

You have to live with your asthma. Control occurs more commonly by learning more about yourself—your personality, character, and lifestyle—and by following your physician's advice, rather than because of any particular medicine he may give you. There is no question that medicine does help. But every day you must make decisions. You live in your own particular environment. In reality, you must treat yourself. If, in this process, you use your physician as your consultant and advisor, and understand fully what you are doing and why you are doing it, the results will be enhanced. Since your physician has skills and greater understanding of asthma and related diseases than you, it is necessary that you work with him regularly. This book is not intended for independent use. While many people with mild asthma buy medications over the counter, I do not advise such an independent course. My goal for you is that, from using this book, and from gaining an increased understanding of your asthma, your need to see your physician for treatment will decrease as you bring your asthma under control.

6

Your Emotional Pattern

Margaret M. was telling me about her daughter, Bobbie.

"Bobbie was crying the other night and I tried to get her to explain why. She had come home alone directly after school because none of the children had asked her to play with them. She had trouble with her homework. By the time she came downstairs for supper, she had begun to have difficulty breathing. After dinner, she went upstairs and started on her homework again. She broke the point on her pencil—and started to cry.

"Hearing her crying, I went to her and asked what was wrong. She said she was having an asthmatic attack. But her breathing wasn't that bad. I knew something else was wrong. Isn't it strange that such a minor thing could cause tears and labored breathing?"

"But what is really minor?" I asked. "Ignored by her friends, upset over her homework, and then a broken pencil point. Did she develop a full-blown asthma attack?"

"No," Mrs. M. replied. "I put my arms around her and got her to tell me about what happened at school. We talked about it a few minutes and before either of us was aware of it, she was fine. She had no attack at all."

A feeling of being unwanted, unloved, and becoming frustrated, triggered Bobbie's breathing problem. Her mother's quick demonstration of love and understanding readily alleviated it. The security of her mother's arms was the most effective medicine that could have been administered. The important point for Bobbie was her mother's quick understanding of the cause of the problem and her instant action to dissipate it.

By pinpointing the cause, one takes the first giant step in circumventing, relieving, or even eliminating the problem.

The questions that follow are designed to help you identify emotional situations that may be factors in your asthma. They include anger and hostility, frustration, fear, sadness, depression, and anxiety. If you identify one or more types of emotional reactions which you can relate to your asthma, the simple *recognition* could be vital. If then, you were to change your handling of a situation, it might free you from an asthmatic attack.

I must point out, however, that it isn't usually as easy to pinpoint problem areas as it was in Bobbie's case. Emotions often overlap each other, and because you may have had an asthmatic attack after you became angry once, does not mean that every time you get angry you are likely to have an asthmatic attack. This is comparable to the psychiatrist who may tell you that he can explain why something happened but cannot always predict when something will occur.

The emotional history questionnaire which follows is designed to help you identify emotional factors or patterns and to develop your understanding of the role emotions may play in your asthma.

Children, of course, cannot answer the same questions adults are asked. Therefore, I have also prepared an "observation" questionnaire for a child. If you are the parent of a young asthmatic, use the observation questionnaire to help evaluate the emotional profile of your child. However, it is difficult to observe one's child objectively. The results may be more accurate if you give the questionnaire to someone else to fill out. Your child's teacher might be a good choice. However, do not inhibit the teacher by asking to see *precisely* how the form was filled out. Instead, just ask in what *category* your child falls, in the teacher's opinion.

While young adults, or anyone else reading this book, may review the observation questionnaire, I would suggest that the adult reader follow the adult questionnaire.

It is difficult to see ourselves clearly—or to see ourselves as others see us. Bobbie Burns said it back in the eighteenth century:

> O wad some Pow'r the giftie gie us
> To see oursels as others see us!

For example a person may *appear* angry to others, but may not *feel* angry himself. What is important, however, is that you identify your emotional and behavioral patterns. Later I will suggest a method which will help you use your findings to alter asthmatic attacks, if your attacks have—in whole or in part—a psychological basis.

For the questionnaires that follow, use the same system you did in filling out your General Medical History form. Prepare a worksheet and label it EMOTIONAL HISTORY WORKSHEET. When the question has a "yes" answer, write down the response, using the capitalized words as a guide. If the answer is "no," go on to the next questions. If you have "no" answers to an entire category, write down "negative" opposite.

OBSERVATION QUESTIONNAIRE FOR CHILDREN

1. Does the CHILD:
   a. Often ACT or seem SELFISH?
   b. DISTURB OTHER children?
   c. ACT QUARRELSOME?
   d. Often TATTLE?
   e. ACT "SMART"?
   f. STEAL?
   g. BULLY OTHER children?
   h. HAVE TEMPER TANTRUMS?
   i. HAVE NO SENSE OF FAIR PLAY?
   j. TEASE OTHER children or INTERFERE WITH THEIR ACTIVITIES?
   k. ACT DEFIANT?
   l. Act IMPUDENT?

    m. Act DESTRUCTIVE?

    n. Appear STUBBORN or UNCOOPERATIVE?

2. Have you noticed that the CHILD OFTEN:
   a. SHOWS POOR COORDINATION?
   b. Is INATTENTIVE?
   c. Has DIFFICULTY CONCENTRATING?
   d. DAYDREAMS?
   e. Appears to be EASILY LED?
   f. Seems to LACK LEADERSHIP?

3. Is the CHILD likely to:
   a. "FALL APART" UNDER STRESS of examination?
   b. Seem OVERSENSITIVE?
   c. Act OVERLY SERIOUS?
   d. Be continuously or frequently SAD?
   e. Be SUBMISSIVE?
   f. Be FEARFUL?
   g. Be OVERLY ANXIOUS TO PLEASE?

4. Does the CHILD often:
   a. SIT FIDDLING with small objects?
   b. HUM OR MAKE OTHER ODD NOISES?
   c. Seem RESTLESS or OVERACTIVE?
   d. Appear EXCITABLE or OVERLY SENSITIVE?
   e. DISTURB, TEASE, or INTERFERE WITH OTHER children?
   f. Excessively DEMAND ATTENTION, especially at school?
   g. Appear OVERLY ANXIOUS to please?

The first set of questions suggests a defiant or aggressive child. Such children tend less to have emotional asthmatic attacks, as they are able to express their anger or hostility. However, if you have noted asthmatic attacks in relation to aggressive behavior, make a special reference to that in your summary on your worksheet.

It is more likely, however, that the more timid, self-reproachful, less manifestly angry person will show a relationship between such behavior and an asthmatic attack. An example: In a "stress test," where asthmatic and non-asthmatic college students were required to perform mental arithmetic while being subjected to verbal criticism *and* time pressure, asthmatic students were inclined to show anxiety, depression, guilt, self-disgust, and shame whereas the "healthy" students became angry and hostile.

The second set of questions tends to characterize a daydreamer, and the third, an anxious, fearful child. The fourth set, which has some overlapping questions, tends to indicate a hyperactive, restless, or even overexcitable, troublesome child. But this category lacks the defiant, aggressive patterns of the first group. If you are having someone fill out the questionnaire in relation to your child, simply ask if your child falls into category 1, 2, 3, or 4.

If your child does not appear to fall into any particular pattern, proceed to the section on allergy.

In the adult questionnaire that follows, you will notice some similarities to the "observation questionnaire." The questionnaire is designed to help you know yourself better in order to reduce to a minimum or even eliminate emotional factors as triggers for asthmatic attacks.

EMOTIONAL HISTORY QUESTIONNAIRE FOR ADULTS

1. *Sadness or Depression Manifestations*:
   a. Are you OFTEN SAD, DEPRESSED, or UNHAPPY?
   b. Do you CRY OFTEN or nearly every day?
   c. Do you WORRY A LOT about personal health, finances, or family problems?
   d. Do you have TROUBLE SLEEPING, falling or staying asleep, or do you want to sleep too much?
   e. Do you USUALLY feel TIRED and EXHAUSTED?
   f. Do you often WISH you were DEAD?
   g. Have you THOUGHT OF COMMITTING SUICIDE or do you have an urge to commit suicide?
   h. Do you OFTEN TAKE A DRINK WHEN THINGS ARE NOT GOING WELL?

2. *Tension and Anxiety Manifestations:*
   a. Do you OFTEN FEEL TENSE?
   b. Do you OFTEN FEEL NERVOUS?
   c. Are there MANY THINGS THAT FRIGHTEN you?
   d. Do you get UPSET EASILY UNDER STRESS?
   e. Are you SENSITIVE AND EASILY HURT by others?
   f. Do you often FEEL your MUSCLES TIGHTEN or your HEART RACE?
   g. Are you AFRAID OF ARGUMENTS?
   h. Do you AVOID DOING, or TRYING, things that you have not done before?

3. *Anger and Hostility Manifestations:*
   a. Do you HAVE FREQUENT ARGUMENTS?
   b. Do you ever BREAK THINGS IN ANGER?
   c. Do you TEND TO "BLOW UP" easily?
   d. Do you DISLIKE BEING CROSSED?
   e. Do you "RAISE A STORM" if you think you're being taken advantage of?
   f. Do you BECOME (UNRULY) ANGRY IF you are KEPT WAITING (with or without cause)?
   g. Do you react angrily and TRY TO GET EVEN if someone else "wins" a contest or event? Or gets a better grade or a job? Or simply if you are disapproved of?
   h. Do you ENJOY "ACTING SMART" or being "A WISE GUY"?
   i. Do you OFTEN STAND UP TO OTHERS, particularly authorities?
   j. Are you STUBBORN about having your own way?

4. *Frustration Manifestations:*
   a. Are you SOMETIMES ANGRY WITH YOURSELF because you did not say what you think you should have said to someone?
   b. Do you OFTEN FEEL you COULD HAVE DONE BETTER or should have acted differently in a certain situation?
   c. Do you TRY TO AVOID COMPLAINTS; try to IGNORE DISCOMFORTS and inconveniences?
   d. Do EMOTIONAL STORMS EXHAUST you?

   e. Do you GET UPSET—AND TRY TO HIDE IT—when a companion makes a scene or asks special favors or foods in a restaurant?

   f. WHEN you ENVY someone do you TEND TO BROOD about it?

   g. Do you OFTEN FEEL INADEQUATE?

   h. Do you feel UNABLE TO EXPRESS OR ASSERT yourself?

   i. Are you WORRIED ABOUT DISAPPROVAL at work or in school?

5. *Fear Manifestations:*

   a. Are you PHYSICALLY AFRAID of injury?

   b. Do you AVOID CONFRONTATIONS BECAUSE you are FRIGHTENED?

   c. Do you seek to AVOID situations where DISAPPROVAL may occur?

   d. Do you feel FEARFUL or PANICKY about SOMEONE or SOMETHING?

Now that you have completed this questionnaire, transfer your positive responses to your worksheet. Does it indicate a pattern of behavior? Check the sample worksheet. It is possible that the variety of your responses does not permit a simple analysis. However, the challenge is to determine whether components of your emotional history are basic causes, or triggers, of your asthma. So, when next you have an attack, sit down and list those incidents which occurred that day. Make a detailed diary. Start with awakening and list, hour by hour, what happened to you until the attack began. If you awoke with an attack, what happened before you went to bed? Did you have a dream? If so, can you recall what it was about? But more important, can you identify how you felt about the various incidents that occurred? Did anything make you angry, upset, frustrated, depressed, or anxious? If any such emotions can be identified, re-read your emotional history and see if you can now identify a pattern. If you can, later you will transfer the information to your Personal Asthma Contract when we begin to list your trigger factors. The sample on the facing page summarizes the data gathered in filling out the emotional history questionnaire.

It may be that emotion is an important factor in your asthma, or a transient one, or it may not be a factor at all. In any event, awareness, self-knowledge, is the key.

SAMPLE EMOTIONAL HISTORY WORKSHEET

Name *John Jones*   Date *Feb. 3, 19—*

Section 1: Often feel sad
             Worry a lot about personal health and family problems
             Usually feel tired and exhausted
Section 2: Feel tense
             Sensitive and easily hurt
             Avoid doing things not done before
Section 4: Often feel could have done better
Section 5: Avoid confrontations because of fear of (verbal) attack
Pattern: Sadness or depression is accentuated when anxious, frustrated, or
           angry.

7

Your Allergic History

A patient remarked to me in the course of discussing probable causes of her asthma that sometimes she thought she was "allergic" to her children.

"An interesting idea," I had responded. I suggested that she consider them antigens and that, under certain circumstances, they provoked an antibody. During those times, she could address them as "allergens." She laughed.

"That's the point," I said. "To laugh about it, to bring the tension to the surface, to avoid getting uptight. When you become tense, your pattern is to develop an asthma attack."

Lord Byron called laughter "cheap medicine." I prefer "best medicine."

The point to remember is that most parents have a "boiling point." It is important for them to recognize when their children's behavior will elicit an excessive response. From a practical point of view, it behooves the parent to cool the atmosphere. A joke can often do it.

Except for the reference to the children as "allergens," this patient story would appear to belong to the chapter on emotions, but often people think they are "allergic" to a member of their family. I have heard an unhappy spouse tell me he thought his asthmatic wife was allergic to him, or vice versa. Perhaps this is, in part, a matter of semantics but the truth is that each asthmatic needs to identify all possible allergens. While in some instances it may be that interpersonal relations play a role, it may also be that one individual carries some allergen that produces bronchospasm in another. My wife, Lora, develops hives when we visit a friend who has a dog. She is allergic to dog saliva. It took some while to detect this.

In this chapter, you, as the detective in your own case of asthma, are called upon to seek out your allergens so that you can avoid them in the future. This is a challenging task. There are two ways to approach it. The first is to study your asthma pattern—the life history of your asthma—to see if there are noticeable clues. The second is to study a long list of common substances to which you might be exposed, or which you might ingest, and see if any stand out as possible causes of your allergy.

There are two other courses also: allergy testing and the "elimination diet." On the latter, you restrict yourself to a few foods that *normally* do not cause allergic reactions and then, after a few weeks or even months, slowly add foods, one at a time, dropping any from your diet that provoke an allergic response.

Even if you undergo allergy testing, the allergist will wish to review your history. Let us see, therefore, if you can isolate some clues as to the characteristics of your asthma pattern. First, you should explore the frequency pattern. Begin a new worksheet. Label it MY ASTHMA PATTERN. Draw a horizontal line and put your present age at the right-hand side of the line and a zero at the left-hand side. If you've had asthma a long time and are not young, you will need to draw a long line. On a one- to five-year basis, mark the line starting with the date of onset of your asthma to the present.

For example, if your asthma started at age 15 and you are now 30 and have had severe, continuing asthma for the past fifteen years, divide the second half of the horizontal line into three five-year periods: 15 to 20; 20 to 25; 25 to 30. (You may also mark the first fifteen years as well.) Now, using a short line for mild periods of attacks and a heavier, longer line to symbolize groups of attacks of greater severity, draw a series of vertical lines in each of those five-year segments. (See sample worksheets on pp. 94–95.)

What you are attempting to achieve is an "at-a-glance" picture of the frequency and severity of attacks during your life span. If your asthma started at age 15, lasted a year, and then did not recur until, say, age 27, chart that pattern.

After you have completed your life pattern, then you must do two additional patterns, as shown in the samples: one for the past year and another for the past month. For the past year, divide the year into quarters, or divide the long horizontal line by thirteen perpendicular lines, indicating each month from January to January. Now, with vertical lines of varying length and weight, indicate the intensity of your asthma during individual months. Use short lines to indicate mild attacks, longer lines to indicate more severe, longer lasting attacks, and heavy, darker lines to indicate very severe periods of asthma.

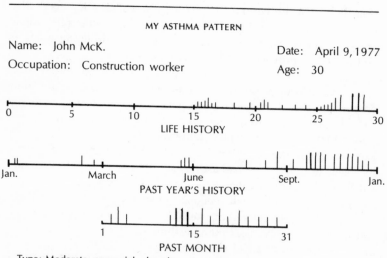

MY ASTHMA PATTERN

Name: John McK.

Date: April 9, 1977

Occupation: Construction worker

Age: 30

LIFE HISTORY

PAST YEAR'S HISTORY

PAST MONTH

Type: Moderate, perennial, chronic.

Note: The winter season, especially if associated with colds, will make this pattern an *intrinsic* type. However, occupation may play a role.

MY ASTHMA PATTERN

Name: Mary C.   Date: February 14, 1977
Occupation: Secretary   Age: 48

LIFE HISTORY

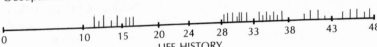

PAST YEAR'S HISTORY

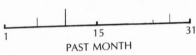

PAST MONTH

Type: Mild, seasonal, acute.
Note: Mary remembered that at age 15 she left the city for the country, and starting at 28, when she married, she moved to the East. Her pattern was clearly *extrinsic*, due to pollens.

MY ASTHMA PATTERN

Name: Peter S.   Date: Nov. 30, 1976
Occupation: Retired banker   Age: 59

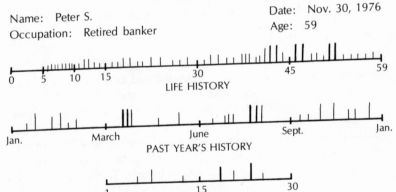

LIFE HISTORY

PAST YEAR'S HISTORY

PAST MONTH

Type: Severe, perennial, chronic.
Note: Although not clearly distinguishable from this chart, the early onset, other signs of allergy (hay fever and family history), and frequent infections clearly indicated a *mixed* type of asthma.

Some months may show no lines at all, indicating a period when you were free of asthma. If your asthma is year-round, the vertical lines will fill up the segment. If your asthma is seasonal, you will have spaces of varying length between the vertical lines as well as differences in the length and weight and number of the lines. You may find that most or all of your vertical lines will be in the spring. In such event, strongly suspect grasses and tree pollens as the source of your asthma. If your asthma occurs in the summer, suspect flowers and ragweed. If your asthma is spotty during the year and is unrelated to colds and infection, suspect dust or molds.

Lastly, plot out the frequency of your asthma during the past month. Again, make a horizontal line and segment it for the weeks. Now, with vertical lines, indicate how often your asthma attacks have occurred. Do you have attacks once a week? Twice a week? Oftener? Daily? Indicate by short lines if the attacks are relatively minor; by longer lines if they are severe. In this way, you and your doctor can review the frequency and severity of your attacks. The chart hopefully will help you identify contact with certain substances during the period of attack, so that you may have clues as to possible allergic components of your asthma.

Evaluation of the severity of attack is the second aspect for you to explore. It will help you measure progress when you have begun your program to control your asthma.

Tommy L., 19, had had severe asthma since his first day in school. When he first became my patient, he had been having almost daily attacks for about a month and had been going to a local emergency hospital once a week and sometimes oftener. Working together, we identified some specific triggers and allergic factors and made charts to indicate the frequency and severity of his asthma, one representing his life since the start of his schooling and onset of asthma, one for the past year, and a detailed one representing his asthma pattern for the previous month. Tommy was started on a regimen to bring his asthma under control.

Three or four weeks later his mother complained: Tommy was still having asthmatic attacks. I questioned both of them about the frequency of the attacks since he had been on the new regimen, and charted Tommy's responses. They watched me as I did it. I then handed Tommy the new chart and the chart I had made the first day I saw him—a chart covering the prior month. They stared at the two charts and were astounded at the difference—the extraordinary reduction in the number of the attacks.

"I never would have believed I could forget so quickly how bad things were," Tommy said. "I'm going to keep these two charts to remind myself."

Your charts will help you do the same. Chart the past month, even if you have had only one asthmatic attack during that period. If that is your regular rate or frequency of attack, consider your asthma very mild. However, if you have had a recent slackening of attacks, that fact alone may indicate that your asthma is occasioned by something unusual or different in the atmosphere.

If you've had four to ten attacks, consider your asthma as moderate, unless all of the episodes were severe. Indicate severity of attack by longer or thicker lines. More than ten attacks during the period constitutes severe asthma.

If your asthma is confined to certain seasons, recognize and describe it as seasonal. If your asthma occurs year-round, describe it as perennial. If you have asthma almost continuously, with minor ups and downs each day and with increasing-decreasing problems of breathing and wheezing, recognize that you have chronic asthma. This is differentiated from intermittent, or acute, asthma. Some chronic asthmatics, however, have frequent acute attacks as well.

On your worksheet, add TYPE OF ASTHMA. Using the checklist on page 98, indicate the type of asthma you have. Later you will transfer the pertinent information to your personal asthma contract. By the time you have completed your analysis of your allergic history, you also should be able to indicate whether your asthma is intrinsic, extrinsic, or mixed.

The process of detecting offending allergens is herculean—and fascinating. It is also essential for control of your asthma. The questionnaire that follows is designed to help you review substances that could initiate an episode of wheezing or gasping for breath.

The questionnaire starts first with some questions about working conditions—even though not all of you are workers. The questionnaire does not encompass all possibilities, but it is intended to

TYPE OF ASTHMA

MILD ☐	MODERATE ☐	SEVERE ☐
SEASONAL ☐		PERENNIAL ☐
ACUTE ☐	INTERMITTENT ☐	CHRONIC ☐
INTRINSIC ☐	EXTRINSIC ☐	MIXED ☐

suggest areas for you to think about so that you may be prompted to recognize possible allergens in your environment. The purpose of the long list is to stimulate your memory about incidents which could involve a substance you may have forgotten about. But whether such a substance is a true allergen for you may require skin testing.

Again, follow the same system as before. In each category, for questions that evoke a "yes" answer, write down the pertinent information on your worksheet, using the capitalized words to help you transfer information. If the answer is "no," go immediately to the next question. If you have no "yes" answers for any one category, write "negative" or "not applicable" on your worksheet, as appropriate.

ALLERGIC HISTORY

1. *Work Environment:*

   At work, are you FREQUENTLY EXPOSED TO:
   a. CHEMICALS, solvents (carbon tetrachloride), etc.?
   b. INSECT KILLERS, plant SPRAYS, or POISONS?
   c. ASBESTOS, CEMENT, GRAIN, COAL DUST?
   d. SANDBLASTING, GRINDING, or ROCK or WOOD dust?
   e. Extreme HEAT?

f. X-RAYS or RADIOACTIVE chemicals?

g. Continuous loud NOISE?

h. Other UNUSUAL SITUATIONS?

If yes, kindly indicate situation(s).

2. *Inhalants:*

a. Are you, or have you been TOLD you are, ALLERGIC TO one or more INHALANTS?

If yes, are you, or have you been told you are, ALLERGIC TO:

b. House DUST?

c. PAINT?

d. GASOLINE fumes?

e. TURPENTINE?

f. BENZINE?

g. RAGWEED?

h. CLOVER?

i. COCKLEBUR?

j. DAHLIA?

k. ELM?

l. GOLDENROD?

m. ORCHARD GRASS?

n. OAK?

o. ROSES?

p. WOOD DUST?

q. MOLD?

r. CAT HAIR?

s. DOG HAIR?

t. RABBIT HAIR?

u. HORSE DANDER?

v. PERFUME?

w. FEATHERS?

x. KAPOK?

y. RAYON?

z. NYLON?

aa. POLYESTER?

bb. SILK?

cc. WOOL?

dd. DETERGENTS?

ee. SOAP?

ff. UNPLEASANT ODORS?

gg. AMMONIA?

3. *Weather Conditions:*

a. Does the CLIMATE, or do CHANGES IN WEATHER, PROVOKE your allergic REACTIONS?

If yes, do you have reactions (WHEEZING, OTHER BREATHING DIFFICULTIES) TO:

b. COLD WIND?

c. DANK WEATHER AND FOG?

d. SUMMER HUMIDITY?

e. SMOG?

f. SNOW?

g. RAIN?

    h. Does your asthma IMPROVE AT THE SEASHORE?

    i. Does your asthma IMPROVE IN DRY DESERT AIR?

    j. Does your asthma IMPROVE IN THE MOUNTAINS?

    k. Does your asthma IMPROVE IN HIGHER ALTITUDES?

4. *Cosmetics and Toiletries:*

    a. Are you, or have you been TOLD you are, ALLERGIC TO one or more COSMETICS and TOILETRIES?

    If yes, are you, or have you been told you are, allergic to:

    b. HAIR DYE?

    c. HAIR SPRAY?

    d. PERFUME?

    e. Underarm DEODORANT SPRAY?

    f. FACE POWDER?

    g. AFTER-SHAVE LOTIONS?

    h. SHAVING CREAM?

    i. BODY LOTIONS?

    j. ORRIS ROOT?

    k. VAGINAL SPRAYS?

    l. OTHER?

    If yes, list offending products or ingredients.

5. *Miscellaneous Everyday Products:*

    a. Are you, or have you been TOLD you are, ALLERGIC TO one or more common, EVERYDAY PRODUCTS?

    If yes, do you have allergic reactions to:

    b. GLUE on POSTAGE STAMPS or ENVELOPES?

    c. NEWSPRINT?

    d. CARDBOARD CONTAINERS for milk, cream, and certain processed juices?

    e. PYRETHRUM (DISINFECTANT)?

    f. INK?

    g. MAGIC MARKERS?

    h. OTHER common products?

    If yes, please list.

6. *Drugs and Chemicals:*
    a. Do you know if you are ALLERGIC TO any DRUGS?
    If yes, do you know if you are allergic to:
    b. ASPIRIN?
    c. PRODUCTS CONTAINING ASPIRIN? (See Aspirin-containing Compounds in the Appendix on pages 181–182.)
    d. ANTIBIOTICS?
    If yes, name which.
    e. COUGH MEDICINE?
    If yes, name KIND and/or INGREDIENTS.
    f. OTHER?
    If yes, specify.

7. *Foods:*
Write down on your worksheet if you are, or strongly suspect you are, allergic to any of the food products listed below. While the list is enormous, fortunately asthma is less commonly due to food factors than to inhalants.

Almonds	Cabbage
Anchovy	Cantaloupe
Apple	Carp
Apricot	Carrot
Arrowroot	Casaba melon
Banana	Cashew
Barley	Catfish
Bass	Cauliflower
Bean (garbanzo)	Celery
Bean (lima)	Cheese (blue)
Bean (soy)	Cheese (Brie)
Bean (string or green)	Cheese (Camembert)
Beef	Cheese (Cheddar)
Beet	Cheese (cottage)
Blackberry	Cheese (goat)
Blueberry	Cheese (Roquefort)
Broccoli	Cheese (Swiss)
Brussel sprouts	Cherry
Buckwheat	Chestnut

Chicken
Chili powder
Chive
Chocolate
Clam
Coconut
Codfish
Coffee
Corn
Cottonseed
Crab
Cranberry
Cucumber
Curry powder
Date
Dill
Distilled beverages:
  Beer
  Wine
  Scotch
  Bourbon
  Rye? Other
Egg
Eggplant
Endive
Fig
Flounder
Garlic
Ginger
Goose
Grape
Grapefruit
Haddock
Halibut
Herring
Honeydew melon
Hops

Horseradish
Kale
Lamb
Leeks
Lemon
Lentil
Lettuce
Lime
Liver
Lobster
Lox
Mackerel
Malt
Mango
Milk (cow)
Milk (goat)
Millet
Mint
Mushroom
Mustard
Nutmeg
Nuts
Oatmeal
Olive (black)
Olive (green)
Onion
Orange
Oregano
Oyster
Papaya
Paprika
Parsley
Pasta (macaroni or spaghetti)
Peach
Peanut
Pear
Peas (black-eyed)

Peas (green)
Perch
Pickerel
Pike
Pimento
Pineapple
Pistachio
Plantain
Plum
Poppyseed
Pork (bacon or ham)
Potato (sweet)
Potato (white)
Prune
Quince
Rabbit
Radish
Raisins
Raspberry
Red snapper
Rhubarb
Rutabaga
Rye flour
Saccharin
Sage
Salmon
Sardine
Sauerkraut
Scallions
Scallop
Sesame
Shad
Shrimp

Smelt
Sole
Soybean oil
Spearmint
Spinach
Squab
Squash
Strawberry
Sturgeon
Sugar (beet)
Sugar (cane)
Swiss chard
Swordfish
Tarragon
Table salt
Tea (black)
Tomato
Trout
Tuna fish
Turbot
Turkey
Turnips
Turtle
Vanilla
Vinegar
Walnut
Watermelon
Wheat
Yam
Yeast (baker's)
Yeast (brewer's)
Zucchini

Sometimes a person is not allergic to a particular food but to an additive intended to make the food look better, taste better, or last longer. In 1976, several additives that have been in use for years were outlawed. However, many foods still contain additives. A few are listed below.

8. *Additives:*

   a. Are you, or have you been TOLD you are, ALLERGIC TO ADDITIVES contained in many commercial foods, including jam, jello, ice cream, jelly, cake, canned goods, etc.?
   If yes, do you have ALLERGIC REACTIONS TO:
   b. MONOSODIUM GLUTAMATE?
   c. METHYLCELLULOSE?
   d. CALCIUM DISODIUM EDTA?
   e. FOOD COLORING?
   f. PHOSPHORIC ACID?
   g. OTHER?
   If yes, specify.

If you have allergies, your allergy worksheet should now resemble the sample that follows. Under suspected allergies, you should have listed first the category, and then the suspicious agent.

When you have completed your allergy history, review it with your medical history and see if you can confirm the type of asthma you have—extrinsic, intrinsic, or mixed. Later, when you see your physician, review your worksheets with him and ask his evaluation of your diagnosis.

At this point you can fill in the date on your Personal Asthma Contract, signifying you have completed the three sections under Specific Knowledge About Myself. You should also indicate the kind of asthma pattern you have (refer to the check list on page 98), if necessary) and you can date that entry too.

Now proceed with a review of your medications history. Save your worksheet, however, because you will need it after you have checked the medications section. It is important to review the section on medications even if you rarely or never use medicines, because knowledge of how drugs work is detailed there.

SAMPLE WORKSHEET
MY ALLERGIC HISTORY

Date: Dec. 3, 19—
Suspected allergies (no tests have been made):

1. *Work Environment:*	Negative
2. *Inhalants:*	House dust
	Perfume
3. *Weather Conditions:*	Hot, sea-level humidity
	Smog
	Cold wind
4. *Cosmetics and Toiletries:*	Soap
	Some hand lotions
	Hair dye
	Hair spray
	Face powder
5. *Miscellaneous Everyday Products:*	Glue on postage stamps and envelopes
6. *Drugs and Chemicals:*	Penicillin
7. *Foods:*	Chocolate
	Nuts
	Yeast
	Shrimp
8. *Additives:*	Monosodium glutamate

MY PERSONAL ASTHMA CONTRACT

Name _____   Date _____

Goal I. Gain Understanding of Asthma   Date Completed

1) General Knowledge   _____

2) Specific Knowledge About Myself   _____
   a) My General Medical History
   b) My Emotional History
   c) My Allergic History

3) My Asthma Pattern:

8

Your Medications History

"Doc," Henry B., a successful businessman in his mid-50s, said to me, "what I really am interested in knowing is how to treat my asthmatic attacks and prevent them. If you tell me I have an allergy, I'll try to avoid those things that cause the problems."

Mr. B., who has had "mild type" asthma for almost thirty years, was saying what a lot of people feel: they want a simple explanation from the physician—instant knowledge about the problem—and an infallible medication.

"My biggest problem," Mr. B. continued, "is knowing what kind of medication to use and when to use it."

"Of course that's the biggest problem," I confirmed. "But in order to select the best medication, you have only two choices: learn through trial and error, or learn through an understanding of what each drug can do."

On that particular day, my next patient had cancelled. Having this unexpected extra time, I asked Mr. B. if he would like to know more about how each of the different asthma medications worked.

"If you think it will help," he responded.

What was interesting to me was that as I began to explain how the different medications produced their effect, it was necessary to review the kind of information I have asked you to gather up to this point. To understand how a medication worked, for example, he needed to know what a cellular reaction was; needed bronchospasm explained; needed a brief understanding of respiration.

Soon Mr. B. began to understand how complex the subject of asthma is and that the more he knew the easier it would be for him to be more selective on his own behalf.

There are hundreds of asthmatic medications on the market. There are so many, in fact, it has been difficult for me to compile a complete list. When I began writing this book, I hoped to be able to provide a chart for you with every over-the-counter medication listed. By doing that, I thought you could review what you might have purchased and examine what your medication was actually doing for you. But the chart I have compiled (see Table 7, Chapter 12) is by no means complete. Even so, you may be surprised to learn that there are really only two actions which a medication can produce to effect bronchodilation, although many have overlapping actions. By that I mean, different drugs may act in more than one way.

Essentially, most medicines either have an action on the cell to prevent formation of some chemical that causes bronchospasm, or an action on the autonomic nervous system, which will cause the bronchial tubes to dilate. Antibiotics, on the other hand, work by destroying bacteria-causing infection. Some medicines, such as antihistamines, or cortisones, have an indirect cellular effect, causing bronchodilation. Table 5 is an attempt to indicate how classes of medications work and their probable site of action. Although antibiotics have been included, they are really non-specific for asthmatics and are indicated only when there is an active infection.

Every class of drugs has a series of side-effects. Since it is not feasible for anyone to attempt to remember all of them, I've listed them in table form so that, should you have any symptoms when you are taking medications, you can refer to the list to see whether or not the symptom might be caused by the medication(s) you are taking. (See Table 6.)

Side-effects from antibiotics are not included because these are

TABLE 5. Action of Medication

Action	Site	Class of Drugs
Anti-bacterial	on bacteria	antibiotics
Anti-spasmodic (Bronchodilator)	on the cell on the autonomic nerves	xanthines adrenalin-like compounds
Anti-allergic	on the cell	antihistamines
Other	mixed or unknown	cromolyn sodium cortisone compounds

medications that should be discussed in detail with the physician who may prescribe them for you. Cortisone is discussed in more detail in Chapter 12.

The route of administration of a medicine—how a medicine enters the body—does not determine where its action takes place or what the action will be. Some medicines are not absorbed well from

TABLE 6. Side-Effects Due to Overdosage

Xanthines	Adrenalin-like Compounds	Antihistamines	Cromolyn Sodium
Nausea	Palpitations and/or irregular pulse	Excessive sleepiness	Sore throat
Fainting			Bronchial irritation
	Headaches		
Flushes			Nasal congestion
	Nervousness or		
Excitation	tremulousness		
Vomiting	Tremors Chest pains		
Irregular pulse			
Irregular heartbeat			

the stomach so that, if taken by mouth, they would be ineffective. This is true of epinephrine or adrenalin, which works best by injection, although it also can work when inhaled in a spray. Most of the antihistamines work well by mouth, as do the antibiotics and cortisone.

Cromolyn works only through inhalation. Medication also can be absorbed via the rectal membranes, and suppositories sometimes are used, especially for children, who may have difficulty swallowing a pill during an acute attack. Children also often have problems inhaling medicines, so that the suppository is an alternate means of administering a drug that might, for an adult, be contained in an inhalant.

With this background, list the current medications you are using or have been using on a fresh worksheet. Make separate lists for those medicines you use for an acute attack, those which you use for allergy, those which you may use if you have an infection, and any other. Put an initial next to each medication to indicate whether you take it by mouth (M), by inhalant spray or aerosol (I), or by suppository (S), and for injections use three initials: INJ.

In Table 5 and the sample worksheet, the term "class of drugs" is used. Class indicates a large group of drugs which act in similar ways. When you check your own medications, you may have trouble learning whether what you are using is a xanthine or an adrenalin-like compound. This is especially true of brand-name drugs because the brand name may not indicate the class and many brands have mixed contents. Phenobarbital, for example, is a common sedative found in tiny doses in many asthmatic compounds. It is used to offset the adrenalin-like action of such medications as ephedrine and Isuprel or vaponephrin which, although different from each other, belong in one class. Penicillin, the mycins—such as erythromycin and the tetracyclines—are all antibiotics. Theophylline, elixophyllin, and aminophyllin are examples of xanthine compounds.

See if you can classify each of the medications you are using. If your medicines are through a doctor's prescription, you may have to call your doctor to ask what they are and how they work. If they are over-the-counter medicines, look at the chemical compound where the contents are listed. See whether you are taking a single medica-

---

SAMPLE WORKSHEET
MY MEDICATIONS HISTORY

Drugs Used For:	*Class (Optional)*
Asthmatic Attack	
a) Tedral (ephedrine) (M)	Adrenalin-like
b) Vaponephrin inhaler (I)	
c) Aminophyllin (S)	Xanthine
Allergy	
a) Chlor-Trimeton (M)	Antihistamine
Infection	
a) Penicillin tablets (M)	Antibiotic
Other	
a) Aarane (I)	Cromolyn sodium

---

tion or one which contains several different compounds. Mixed medications frequently are found in over-the-counter preparations and you may have to do a little detective work if the contents listed do not appear in the list provided for you in Chapter 12.

If you want to break down your over-the-counter drugs into classes, ask your pharmacist for help. He can tell you immediately into which class the drug falls and may also help you in connection with prescription drugs.

Before you start your medications worksheet, check the sample at the top of this page. After you fill out your worksheet, add a new subheading to your Personal Asthma Contract, "My Medications History." Under that subheading, list your current medications classified under the four headings "Asthmatic Attack," "Allergy," "Infection," and "Other"—if you are taking other medications. Your contract should then look like the sample that follows.

MY PERSONAL ASTHMA CONTRACT

Name _____   Date _____

Goal I. Gain Understanding of Asthma   Date Completed

  1) General Knowledge   _____

  2) Specific Knowledge About Myself   _____
     a) My General Medical History
     b) My Emotional History
     c) My Allergic History

  3) My Asthma Pattern: _____

  4) My Medications History for: _____

     a) Asthmatic Attack

     b) Allergy

     c) Infection

     d) Other

9

Putting It All Together

By now, some factors in your asthma ought to be fairly apparent. Check over your worksheets for those factors which you know, or suspect, may be related to asthma. Note possible trigger factors, or conditions, that may require further investigation by a physician. On your Personal Asthma Contract add another new subheading: "Trigger Factors," and under it, four columns titled "General," "Emotional," "Allergic," and "Other." Leave adequate space for all the items you may want to draw from your various worksheets to list as trigger factors. The sample contract that follows illustrates the kind of information that should be present up to this point.

Should your history suggest a condition that might be important but appears unrelated to your lungs or your asthma, make a special note to be sure to check out this condition with your physician when you next see him.

The purpose of the list is to force you to create an increased awareness of those conditions which are likely to start an asthmatic attack. Avoidance of these initiating factors will be an important aspect of control of your asthma.

MY PERSONAL ASTHMA CONTRACT

Name: Fred S.

Date: Dec. 1, 19--

Goal I. Gain Understanding of Asthma   Date Completed
  1) General Knowledge   Dec. 1
  2) Specific Knowledge About Myself   Dec. 6
    a) My General Medical History
    b) My Emotional History
    c) My Allergic History
  3) My Asthma Pattern:
    CHRONIC, PERENNIAL, MODERATELY SEVERE, MIXED   Dec. 6
  4) My Medications History for: Dec. 12
    a) Asthmatic Attack
        MARAX
        ISUPREL SPRAY
        ADRENALIN when severe
    b) Allergy
        SHOTS
        CHLOR-TRIMETON
    c) Infection
        ERYTHROMYIN
    d) Other
        VALIUM
  5) Trigger Factors: Dec. 15
    a) General
        COLD AIR
        HEAVY POLLUTION
    b) Emotional
        WHEN BEHIND IN WORK
        WHEN WIFE SPENDS TOO MUCH MONEY
    c) Allergic
        DUST
        MOLD
        YEAST
        ASPIRIN
        PENICILLIN
    d) Other
        COLDS

What Can Be Done and
What You Should Expect

10

What Can the Doctor Do?

A young singer came to my office with the beginning of a laryngitis. He had been working hard and had noted a slight hoarseness over the previous few days. I examined him and said he might be developing a mild cold but that I wasn't certain.

"What can you do?" he asked.

"I don't think *we* should do anything," I replied.

"You mean you don't have some injection, spray, or pill that I can take?" he queried.

When I shook my head, he said, perhaps jokingly, or perhaps seriously, "Gee, Doc! What good are you?"

The answer is that a doctor possesses knowledge of things to do under many circumstances and of things not to do in many others. Frequently a "wait and see" period of caution, observation, and restrictive therapy is indicated.

In the course of this book, you have been examining what is happening when you have an asthma attack and why it is happening. You have begun to look at what you can do to help yourself, with the help of your doctor, of course. You have gathered data about yourself and have begun to learn what kind of asthma you have. This is the first step toward diagnosis and definition of your treatment program. But an accurate diagnosis may require testing before establishment of any new treatment program.

It is now time to plan an appointment with your doctor to review your histories with you; confirm whether you have an intrinsic, extrinsic, or mixed asthma; determine the amount of infection—if any—that may be superimposed on your asthma; and find out if there are any additional factors that may be contributing causes. A general physical checkup would be an excellent idea.

If you go to your physician when your asthma has subsided, your physical examination should be entirely normal, unless you have other diseases or complications. When your doctor listens to your heart and lungs and takes your blood pressure, you should be no different from any other reasonable healthy person. On the other hand, if your general medical history outlines possible complaints related to the heart, lungs, intestinal or urinary tract, or some other problem, your doctor will decide, in conference with you, whether you should have additional examinations and tests. Should there be other problems, use the four basic questions I suggested earlier: What is happening? Why is it happening? What can *we* do about it? What can I expect?

SPECIAL TESTS

By now, in relation to your asthma, you probably will have decided whether you have specific emotional problems or allergies, but there may also be evidence of other complications. This is likely to be true if you have long-term chronic asthma where combinations of infection and recurring bronchitis become associated with emphysema. Sometimes this can be ascertained from the physical examination alone. For example, your chest expansion may be a clue. If your chest expansion is less than one inch at the nipple line and you know it used to be much more, you should be checked for the possibility of emphysema. But your chest expansion should never be measured during a wheezing episode because it is likely to be restricted at such a time.

Another test that your doctor might do is one I like to call the "huff" test. You can do this test yourself. Light a match and hold it about three inches from your mouth. Holding your mouth *wide open*, "huff" out the match with air from your *lungs*. Do not take in new air to "huff" out the match. Since asthmatics and emphysematous patients have difficulty exhaling air from their lungs, they often are unable to "huff" out the match.

To confirm or deny the possibility of emphysema or other complications, your doctor may request a chest X-ray and/or an electrocardiogram—the latter for adult asthmatics only. As a rule, it is uncommon for children to require special heart examinations.

Some patients ask me about blood tests but there are no blood tests which are helpful in asthma, although the blood count—and the sputum—may sometimes show a special cell called an eosinophil in people who have allergy. However, doctors rarely test for this cell.

If infection is considered likely, the most important test is a sputum culture. From testing the sputum, the doctor learns what specific germs are present in the mucus and which antibiotic will be most effective. Allergy studies also may be recommended.

While sometimes it may seem that the science of medicine has been baffled by asthma, there has been an enormous amount of research and study in the last several years about pulmonary and chest diseases. This research has produced a variety of important studies and tests, which frequently are recommended for some asthmatics and others with chronic lung disease. These tests can aid greatly when certain kinds of asthma come to the doctor's attention. Specifically, there are special breathing tests which determine causes and defects in air passage and transportation of oxygen to the bloodstream.

To review two of these tests:

The first test measures *vital capacity*. The vital capacity is the amount of air which you take in when you inhale deeply and the amount of air which is expelled when you breathe out as fully as possible. This inspiration and expiration—the respiratory cycle—is measured by breathing into a special machine. From your size and weight, it is known what your "normal" capacity should be. Asthmatics, of course, may have a decreased vital capacity, although mild asthma sufferers may be able to breathe normal amounts of air in and out. They just take much longer to do it.

The second test measures *timed vital capacity*. The timed vital capacity is the amount of air which can be expired—breathed out—in one second. It is essentially like the "huff" test, but graphically demonstrates the delay in passage of air through the narrowed bronchial tubes that occurs during asthmatic attacks. Other breathing tests are available but these are performed for special reasons only and on the recommendation of your doctor.

Once you have classified your asthma and found out the general state of your lungs, it is time to determine the kind of treatment control your asthma requires. That means it is time to look at some of your options. Let's start with an interesting one: solving allergic problems.

ALLERGY TESTING

As an internist, when I recommend a consultation with another physician, people almost always are appreciative. But there are two kinds of doctors where a great deal of persuasion may be required before patients are ready to accept their services. The first is the psychiatrist. Typical patient responses:

"I don't need a psychiatrist!"

"You think there's something wrong with my head?"

"I don't want to see a shrink!"

The second doctor who evokes patient protest is the allergist. The response is usually:

"All those needles!"

To test for allergies, the allergist places the potential allergic material just underneath the outer layers of the skin. If you're allergic, the skin swells around it and ordinarily turns red so that the response is readily seen. This is called a positive reaction. If you are not allergic to that particular allergen, there is no reaction, which is called a negative reaction. Identification of your allergies by skin testing can be complicated by the fact that your allergic manifestation may be due to substances other than those you are being tested for. However, when you know at least some of the things your skin reacts to and have taken a careful history, you can begin to make certain deductions. But even then, it's complicated. For example, allergy to penicillin occurs frequently, but unfortunately a skin test is not a reliable method of determining whether an allergy to penicillin exists. You can have a positive reaction with a skin test and never react adversely to penicillin medication at all, or you can have a negative skin test reaction and have a severe penicillin allergy—or even a shock reaction. The same is true of many other substances.

Shock reaction during allergy testing, or anaphylaxis, I might add, is uncommon. However, in case it might occur, the allergist always has a syringe full of adrenalin handy to counteract any such situation. You truly need not worry about this kind of response, and you needn't worry about the needles hurting. Few people find that tests are painful.

The number of tests required for reliable diagnosis depends largely upon the individual. Suspected allergens are tested for first. Once you come to food allergens, though, a large number of tests could be required. But it should be kept in mind that adults are not likely to have asthmatic reactions to foods, although children often do. With most adults, molds, dusts, and pollens are usually the offenders.

If testing determines that you are allergic to a particular food, the simple solution is: avoid the food. If it's dust or molds, you may have to create a dust-free environment for yourself. If you are shown to be allergic to pollens—trees and grasses—the answer may be a series of desensitizing shots. The purpose of such injections is to reduce the sensitivity to the substance to which you are allergic. For example, if you're a hay fever sufferer living in a climate where ragweed grows abundantly, shots can be recommended to reduce your sensitivity to ragweed. This is done by giving injections of ragweed itself—very tiny doses at first and building up to a substantial dose that becomes the maintenance injection. The maintenance is continued for an indefinite period of time. If there is a seasonal allergy, the dose is increased in frequency during the season when the person is likely to be allergic and decreased during the rest of the year—perhaps to once a month or every six weeks.

If you prove to be allergic to a lot of foods, the easiest thing is to start with an elimination diet, where you forego all the foods suspected of causing allergies. After a few days—a minimum of a week and sometimes up to three—on a very simple, easily digested diet, you slowly add foods—one at a time. In this way you may identify those foods you can eat, even if skin tests have shown you to be allergic to that food. It is important that the diet be varied and that suspected foods be eaten only intermittently, so as to be certain of the reaction. If a food that is added to the diet does cause an adverse reaction, it should be eliminated from the diet permanently. In children, elimination diets may be tried instead of using skin tests. (See Appendix.)

If dust is a serious cause of allergy for you, then it may be necessary to create a dust-free environment. (See Appendix.)

If tests show a need to improve your breathing, you should include breathing exercises in your program, or take up playing a wind instrument, or blow up balloons two or three times a day. The Appendix contains breathing exercises.

It is now time to create a second section of your Personal Asthma Contract, which is for your second goal: "Develop Prevention Program." Under prevention, first you need to list "Physician Consultation." When you talk with your doctor and he reviews your history, discuss with him whether you should have special tests and whether there may be an allergic component in your asthma. If there is a suspicion of allergy, your doctor may recommend allergy tests. Note what additional tests the doctor may recommend and indicate on your Personal Asthma Contract when they are completed.

Next on your contract, you need to list "Allergy Prevention." If allergy is not a factor in your asthma, write "not indicated." But if allergy is present, then there may be several subsections that you will have to include, such as desensitization, dust-free environment, or establishment of an elimination diet. (See following sample.)

By now, you realize that good health requires more than simply putting yourself into the hands of a good doctor. There is much that only you can do, and that's the subject of the next chapter: Things you can do for yourself.

Goal II. Develop Prevention Program   Date Completed

1) Physician Consultation: _____

   a) "Histories" Review   _____

   b) Additional Examinations   _____

      Physical examination   _____

      Special breathing tests   _____

      Blood tests   _____

      X-rays   _____

      EKG   _____

      Allergy studies   _____

2) Allergy Prevention: _____

   a) Create dust-free environment   _____

   b) Plan an elimination diet   _____

   c) Desensitization   _____

11

Things You Can Do for Yourself

Mark G. is an actor who loves to play the violin. If you see him in an acting role carrying a fiddle case, you can expect there will be a gun inside, since Mark often is cast in the role of a gangster. In spite of the fact that he looks the gangster part as well as acts it, he is a gentle soul. His wife, Barbara, is equally gentle. Barbara was visiting one day shortly before they were to leave for California with their son, Keith, who is the asthmatic in the family.

"Mark has a series of parts to do and they're being filmed in Los Angeles," Barbara told me. "We're taking Keith with us and we'll be in the Los Angeles area over the summer. What do you think it will be like for Keith and his allergies out there?"

"Los Angeles has more than a fair amount of pollution which could cause him some discomfort," I replied, "but if he is faithful taking his medication, he should not have any real problem."

"What about his immunization shots?" she asked.

I thought for a minute. "Have you ever considered giving them to him yourself? Keith is on a stable dose and I'm sure your allergist would teach you how to give the injections."

"Could I do that?" she asked. "But I don't much like the idea of jabbing Keith with a needle."

We talked a few moments, and Barbara agreed to ask her allergist. The allergist, recognizing that the immunization shots for Keith were like a fixed dose of insulin that a diabetic quickly learns to administer to himself, thought the suggestion a good one. He taught Barbara how to measure the dose and adjust the disposable syringe to get rid of any air bubble. He recommended that she administer Keith's weekly shot on the same day of the week and at about the same hour so as to make the shots as routine as possible.

Except for a few episodes of asthma when the smog was particularly bad, Keith did well that summer. Barbara's role in administering shots to Keith set me to thinking about the idea that patients could give themselves not only their immunization shots for allergy but perhaps even adrenalin injections when necessary. The question of how much a patient should do for himself began to seem increasingly worthy of further investigation.

When a patient learns about his own capabilities, he becomes much more free. He can travel, for instance, without worrying about what he can do about his allergy shots. Sending an asthmatic or allergic child off to camp with his doctor's instructions to a camp nurse about frequency and dosage is routine once desensitization has been completed. The more an asthmatic—adult or child—learns how to control his asthma himself, the less frightening the disease appears; therefore, the more readily it can be controlled.

When dust is implicated as a prime cause of an allergic reaction, the asthmatic—adult or child—should sleep in a dust-free environment. On first thought, the creation and maintenance of a dust-free room may seem terribly challenging. But it can be managed without difficulty once you can bring yourself to establish a sleeping room that has the austerity of a monk's cell.

Mary Ann, one of our office nurses, who is an asthmatic strongly allergic to dust, said she found that the smaller the room, the easier the task. A basic decision must be made to eliminate draperies, wool carpeting, upholstered chairs and couches, any such decorative devices as a canopied, four-poster bed, books, and even framed paintings and photographs. A child's room should contain a minimum of toys and all should be washable.

There are two kinds of dust—that which seeps through the windows from city streets, which can be mopped up or dusted away, and the kind of dust that accumulates in mattresses, pillows, clothing, upholstered furniture, and stuffed toys. (Detailed instructions for creating a dust-free environment are contained in the Appendix.)

As you consider all the other things you can do to help bring your asthma under control, check the following subjects for clues.

FATIGUE

Prevent states of exhaustion. Learn to give up "compulsive work" habits and stop working when fatigue sets in. Excessive fatigue, mental or physical, from work or play, can encourage an asthma attack and emergence of repressed allergies.

Avoid carrying too-heavy packages and suitcases.

Get enough sleep.

A good rule is: If you begin to feel tired, you've already done too much.

CLIMATE AND AIR POLLUTION

Be aware of reactions to climate. When hot, humid weather is a trigger, try to avoid it, or reduce activity as much as possible. If you live in a continuously hot, humid area, consider moving to a different climate. However, while some who have moved from sea-level northeastern states to high-altitude Colorado or dry southern Arizona have been benefited by the change, others making similar drastic moves—giving up jobs and selling their homes—have found their asthma as bad if not worse in the different climate. A one-time visit is not sufficient evidence on which to decide whether a climate change will be of benefit. Some who make moves to other states and countries and do benefit attribute their improvement to the difference in climate. Sometimes, however, the real reason for the improvement is absence of a particular kind of stress that existed in the old environment—a situation, or perhaps a person.

It's a cliche that no one can do anything about the weather, but it's not precisely true. There are a variety of steps an asthmatic can take to help reduce or eliminate weather-induced triggers for asthmatic attacks.

For instance, when an inversion occurs—that is, when the air becomes stagnant and a large amount of dust or chemical contaminants accumulate—the asthmatic should stay indoors as much as possible. He should reduce his activity or, at the very least, avoid any unnecessary physical strain during periods of heavy air pollution.

A person with chronic bronchitis is particularly likely to be affected when the atmosphere contains a lot of sulphur fumes.

An air filtering device on an air conditioner may be helpful. Other asthmatics, particularly those with more complicated lung disease, may do well to rest in bed or in a chair until the inversion passes.

CLOTHING

When affected by heat or cold, or both, the asthmatic should pay special attention to mode of dress so as to be as cool as possible in summer. In cold weather, keep head, hands, and feet well protected. Wear a hat and gloves. If cold wind and air trigger an attack for you, cover your mouth and nose loosely with a scarf and walk as little as possible outdoors on a cold, windy, wintry day.

FOOD

In addition to avoiding known food allergens, eat moderately and slowly. One of my asthmatic patients told me that she had been teaching herself to eat more slowly by putting her fork or spoon on her plate between mouthfuls.

"It's astonishing how that little trick helps," she said. "Now that I've slowed down, I find I eat less and am more relaxed. In fact, meal time for the entire family has become much more relaxed and enjoyable."

Adequate fluids are essential for the asthmatic. Water is almost as important as a medication. During a severe attack, force the water intake to far more than six to eight glasses for the day. Don't worry about food intake. Most asthmatics find it difficult to eat very much, if anything, during an attack.

CONSTIPATION

While there is no reliable research relating toxic body wastes to asthma, an asthmatic can be particularly uncomfortable if dehydrated and unable to eliminate. Drinking lots of water and eating plenty of fruits and vegetables and other roughage such as bran are the simplest measures to ensure adequate elimination. Avoid laxatives unless your physician specifically prescribes one. Natural bran found in health food stores is often more effective than the commercial all-bran cereals.

EXERCISE

Asthma is a handicap, and recurring asthma frequently puts a limitation on certain kinds of exercise and physical activity. However, there are many sports open to the asthmatic and studies show that a number can be helpful. Swimming, tests show, increases breathing abilities as well as providing superior all-around exercise.

General rules to follow in relation to children:

1. Physical training and physical education within the peer group is recommended except for those with severe asthma. Asthmatics often feel that both diaphragm and chest muscle training and general conditioning decrease wheezing. Learning to play a wind instrument may be extremely helpful.

2. The use of a bronchodilator ten to fifteen minutes before activity may be advisable, particularly for those who normally develop wheezing on exertion. Sometimes a dose after exercise may also be necessary.

3. Activities which require short bursts of energy—one to two minutes at a time—are more desirable than those which require steady, prolonged, strenuous exertion.

4. While swimming is the "best" sport for asthmatics, badminton, softball, ping pong, archery, bowling, and golf generally are well tolerated. Football, running, tennis, basketball, and handball usually are too strenuous.

5. During periods when asthmatic attacks have recurred because of season, weather, infection, pollution, or for other reasons, arrangements should be made for the asthmatic in school to be assigned alternate activities and to be excluded from physical competition that could be embarrassing.

6. In today's competitive sports, the asthmatic taking medication must report drugs used and conform to the rules about medications consistent with the sport.

While I and other doctors urge extreme moderation in use of bronchodilation inhalers, use of the medication before exercising—even before such breathing exercises as you find in the Appendix—can be helpful. The asthmatic teen-age daughter of one of my patients always puts a bronchodilator spray into her purse when she goes out dancing. She is relaxed about her problem and her friends respect her for it. None of her friends teases if she stops dancing to use the spray and rest. She is well aware of problems of overusage. Having learned to use it properly, she never feels it necessary to use it oftener than once in four hours. Each of her friends is eager to give supportive help if she does have an attack and none ever suggests leaving her home because of her "problem."

COLDS

The best way to handle a cold is not to get one. It's sensible to stay away from crowded places during times when colds seem very prevalent. However, it is extremely difficult to prevent all upper respiratory infections, so flu vaccine is a good idea for most asthmatics.

At the first sign of a cold or other infection, the asthmatic should stay at home—in bed, if possible. Bed rest protects the sufferer from overexertion, changes in temperature, and, generally, from stress.

(Hopefully, the bed will be in a dust-free room. Keep the door closed to prevent any irritating odors from entering the bedroom from other areas of the home.)

Ask your physician for an expectorant cough mixture which you can keep on hand to be used at the first sign of a chest cough. Repeat every four hours as necessary to control the cough. The cough mixture may help loosen phlegm in the bronchial tree and enable the asthmatic to cough up mucus more easily. Using a humidifier has not proven to be effective regularly. In fact, some asthmatics may worsen with use of a humidifier. The rule is: Try it. If you like it, use it. If not, use other measures.

Drink at least six to eight glasses of water daily and plenty of juices too. In children, restrict food to the amount that is comfortably tolerated. Serve hot broth, small servings of chicken or easily digested meat and vegetables. Take the temperature morning and evening and note it on a sheet of paper, along with a listing of medications given, time they are given, and the food and liquids ingested.

If there is no improvement after twenty-four hours, or a severe asthmatic attack has occurred, call your physician. He must check to determine if antibiotic drugs may be necessary. Following these simple remedies, eliminating as many other triggers as possible, having your doctor find and remove hidden infections, and using antibiotics wisely, are the best ways to prevent an infectious component that could be the cause of your asthma.

SMOKING

Elimination of smoking can be one of the most important aspects of an asthmatic's treatment program. If you are addicted to cigarettes, it won't be easy, but with good health as your goal, it's absolutely necessary.

Giving up cigarettes will benefit you and your entire family—and help your pocketbook too. Research shows that in the majority of families where parents don't smoke, the children tend not to smoke either. Studies suggest that smoking in the home adversely affects the non-smokers too. A 19-year-old patient of mine, who had severe, chronic asthma, showed marked improvement when her father stopped smoking.

The major cause of chronic lung disease is cigarette smoking. Inhalation of cigarette smoke, and other pollutants, affects one of your important lung defenses—the cilia. Cilia are tiny hairs—tens of millions of them—along your air passages. They wave back and forth, normally about twelve times a second. Under a microscope, they make you think of a field of grass waving in a steady, gentle breeze.

It's the job of the cilia to sweep out particles before they penetrate deep into the lungs. Cigarette smoking slows down their action. Through irritation of the bronchial tubes, susceptibility to infections and accumulation of mucus increases. Smoke can paralyze and destroy the normal cilia activity.

Cigarette smoke—and other air pollutants—also constrict the air passages, making breathing more difficult. These pollutants reduce the efficacy of the scavenger cells, the macrophages, in the lungs, whose purpose is to eat up invading substances. Even one puff of a cigarette can slow down the activity of the macrophages in an asthmatic.

A very real benefit enjoyed by non-smokers: fewer develop emphysema. Except for a tiny percentage of people born with a certain enzyme deficiency, most persons who develop emphysema have been heavy smokers for years. Anyone who smokes increases the likelihood of being affected by chronic bronchitis and emphysema, arteriosclerosis, lung cancer, heart disease, stroke, and perhaps other conditions. Put bluntly: Cigarette smoking reduces life expectancy.

Milton R. is Director of the Audio-Visual Department of the American Lung Association. The Association's interest in the American public's smoking habits is well known. Their slogan, "it's a matter of life and breath," has been used extensively to emphasize their anti-smoking program. "Stanley," Milton said to me after reviewing this section, "you must say more than you have to convince the asthmatic that he must give up smoking."

But what else can I say? You know what you must do. The important thing is that you must act.

Some years ago shortly after I had started practice, a young man came to me with a bad bronchitis. He said he had tried to stop smoking many times and failed. Would I hypnotize him? When we discussed the pros and cons, I told him that if he really wanted to stop he could do so without hypnotism.

He insisted and so I tried. He was an excellent subject; he followed my suggestions and rapidly fell into a deep trance. I suggested that when he awakened he would feel normal and would not want to smoke. But then I added that if he did smoke the cigarette would taste like burning celluloid and that he would become nauseated. This post-hypnotic suggestion, I told him, would continue for a week. Then I awakened him.

He told me he felt fine, and he remembered my instructions. I asked him to call for an appointment for the following week and we would proceed according to his needs.

About three weeks later I reminded myself that he had not returned. Curious, I called his office to ask what had happened. I have never forgotten his reply. In fact it convinced me never to use hypnosis again.

"It was a very interesting experience," he said. "When I arrived home I suddenly remembered what you had said about cigarettes tasting different. I noticed that I had no desire to smoke, but I was curious to see what would happen. I lit up and the taste was awful. I couldn't smoke because I became nauseous.

"After dinner, I just had to try it again. I couldn't believe what I had experienced. I opened a fresh pack and lit up. It was just as bad. I tried again before I went to sleep and it was the same. The next morning I noticed that the bad taste was a little less nauseating. Doc, do you know it took me a week before I could get rid of that lousy taste?"

I never saw him again. Need I say more?

Thus to the prevention program of your Personal Asthma Contract, I urge you to add—if you are a smoker—"Stop smoking." You also may wish to add two other headings, the first of which relates to establishing a procedure for air pollution or inclement weather and for upper respiratory infection (colds), and the second to planning a breathing and general exercise program. Your asthma prevention program is now complete and that part of your Personal Asthma Contract should be like the following sample.

The next chapter deals with medications so that you will be able to gain greater understanding of the options available to you and develop a treatment plan for regular use.

Goal II. Develop Prevention Program	Date Completed
1) Physician Consultation:	_____
a) "Histories" Review	_____
b) Additional Examinations	_____
Physical examination	_____
Special breathing tests	_____
Blood tests	_____
X-rays	_____
EKG	_____
Allergy studies	_____
2) Allergy Prevention:	_____
a) Create dust-free environment	_____
b) Plan an elimination diet	_____
c) Desensitization	_____
3) Stop Smoking	_____
4) Establish Procedure for:	_____

　　a) Air Pollution or Inclement Weather　　　　　_____

　　b) Upper Respiratory Infection　　　　　　　　_____

5. Establish Breathing and General Exercise Program　　_____

12

What You Should Know About Medications

When I write a prescription for a medication, I am prescribing what I believe will best benefit the patient, but in no illness is the patient's participation required more than in asthma. There are many options. What works for one may not for another. Therefore, when you review your own medications history and consider the alternatives open to you, keep in mind the overall goal to control your asthma and prevent attacks.

A professor of mine once remarked, "There are no good drugs. Only good doctors." What he was implying is that drugs are foreign to the body. You are better off without any. Certainly you should take none if you are in good health. But, as an asthmatic, you aren't, so the goal must be to take the minimum amount of medication necessary to achieve control, and to take it as instructed.

I often assume that the patient will follow the prescribed treatment correctly, yet I also *know* that most patients hope that the illness will simply go away—as though by some kind of miracle.

Patients fall into different categories. The optimistic patient is sometimes the one who is the worst about following through and taking
the medications that have been prescribed and bought. The op-
timist falls into a group I call the ostriches. He feels it is best if he
takes no medicine or as little as possible, hoping, or making believe,
the asthma will miraculously cease.

Another type has trouble remembering to take his medications.
He is conscientious, but when he has no symptoms, he often
forgets.

"How do you remember to take the pills?" a patient of mine once
asked. Then he joked, "I often am so active I forget all about it. How
do you remember to remind yourself when you don't remember?"

This problem of remembering is especially difficult if a medication is taken to prevent rather than to treat. It's easy to remember to
take a pill when you are having trouble breathing, but to prevent an
attack when you're busy doing other things—well, that's another
matter.

Often physicians try to link pill-taking with a regular activity, such
as meals. If pills are taken before meals when the stomach is empty,
they usually are absorbed fairly rapidly and their effect takes place
more quickly than when taken on a full stomach. Hence, doctors
make a decision as to whether they want rapid action or delayed and
longer action from a pill. In any case, they are apt to advise you to
take medications at mealtime. For example, if you are told to take a
pill every morning, an easy way to remember is to take it with your
juice at breakfast.

Another method that I have found to be useful is to develop an
absurd mental association. If you create a silly mental picture in
association with something you do regularly, your memory will be
aided greatly. For example, some people don't eat breakfast but
may only grab a cup of coffee on the run. It wouldn't be practical for
them to try to take a pill as they rush out the door. Most people,
however, do brush their teeth in the morning. Keeping the pills
next to the toothbrush and mentally conjuring up an enormous pill
imbedded in the bristles of your toothbrush is a good way to create a
habit. The giant pill should be the same color and shape as the one
you are required to take, except multiplied in size many times over.

The silly picture of the huge pill on the little toothbrush is something that is hard to forget. Of course, once the habit is well developed, you won't need the image at all.

Another "silly picture": Imagine your alarm clock as a giant pill so that, when it goes off in the morning, you will see it as a pill—and remember to take your medication.

Reading the morning paper at the breakfast table is a habit of millions of Americans. Picture a bottle of pills falling from the newspaper as you open it—and rolling right toward you, ready for you to open the cap and pop one into your mouth. I am sure you can think of more pertinent examples related to things you commonly do everyday. To sum up, remember by associating. Associate your required medications with something that is familiar and routine and develop a mental picture that is unusual.

THE TREATMENT PROGRAM

Asthmatics often require many different kinds of medication. You have already listed medications which fall into four categories. These include regular asthmatic medications, those for allergy, those for infection, and other. It is important that we examine the different kinds of pills, liquids, inhalants, suppositories, and injections and the principles of their action in order to help you and your physician develop the best medications plan for you. I say you *and* your physician because, while your doctor can help you choose a medication, only you will know from your own experience which medication helps you breathe best.

CONTINUOUS BRONCHODILATION

To begin, let us analyze the need for medications which prevent bronchial spasm, or, to put it another way, which dilate the bronchial tubes. Easy breathing requires your bronchial tubes be as wide open as possible at all times.

Take a worksheet and label it MY TREATMENT PROGRAM. (See

samples on pages 157–158.) On the left-hand side, put a new heading: "Continuous Bronchodilation." Under this heading you will list drugs which prevent bronchial spasm. For some of you, there is no need for continuous bronchodilation. You are among the lucky ones who have intermittent short episodes of spasm. In such case, you would write "not indicated" under the heading, and reserve your listings for one or both of the other headings we will discuss later in this chapter.

If you are a person with an allergy that is controlled by use of a simple antihistamine daily, you would list the antihistamine under the "continuous" heading and then you too would be finished with this section.

For a great many asthmatics, however, the daily routine for prevention of bronchospasm requires complex treatment. An antihistamine may be ineffective in relation to the goal of continuous bronchodilation. If you use an antihistamine at all, it might be only occasionally and, if so, you would list this drug under one of the other column headings you will be directed to add later.

Any drug you are taking daily, list for simplicity's sake under the "continuous" heading. If you are taking a medication currently and are not sure whether or not you should be taking it daily, check with your physician. When we complete these columns, your treatment plan will be one of the very important matters for you to review with your doctor, both to prevent any possible misunderstanding and also because, in your case, he may have some special recommendations. A most important aspect of this medication plan will be a recognition of *your understanding* of how you use each of your medicines and what they are being used for.

The first group of drugs which produce continuous bronchodilation are the *ephedrine* compounds. Most over-the-counter asthma medications contain one of the ephedrine group and, in fact, often contain additional medications as well. On page 142 you will find a list of medications which you should use to check the contents of drugs that you have been taking. If one contains ephedrine, be sure to list it under the "continuous" heading.

Ephedrine belongs to the adrenalin-like class of drugs which, technically, are called adrenergic or sympathomimetic drugs. Many of this class, especially ones that work well by pill form, can be used to create a continuing bronchodilation by stimulation of the sympathetic nerves. An easy way to remember this fact is by keeping in mind that the sympathetic nerves are also called adrenergic nerves. The word *adrenergic* resembles *adrenalin*. Remember that adrenalin also is called epinephrine. Ephedrine is chemically different from epinephrine, but works the same way. There is an adult-size ephedrine pill and a pediatric size—to ensure that children are not overmedicated. Too much of the medication has a tendency to produce nervousness and shaking of the limbs or other signs of stimulation. (See Table 6, page 109.) For this reason, phenobarbital often is used with ephedrine. Put simply: Adrenalin and epinephrine are the same thing but ephedrine is different. However, the two drugs act through the same part of the nervous system to cause bronchodilation.

The ideal medicine would cause the maximum dilation with no other effects. But since the sympathetic nerves transmit messages to the blood vessels, the intestines, and the bladder as well as the bronchial tubes, when you stimulate the nerves to achieve bronchodilation, you stimulate other things too. These other stimulations are called "side-effects." We doctors are always looking for a medicine which limits its effects to just one area.

Some people can take a lot of ephedrine and not be bothered. Others can't. What I want you to understand, though, is that you may need to find a medication which you can take three or four times a day without side-effects in order to produce a continuing bronchodilation when you need it. The adrenergic group of drugs may do this for you. Keep in mind that *twenty-four-hour bronchodilation* is the goal. The medication or medications which achieve this for you should be listed under the "continuous" heading. I say medications because often it may be that you will need to take more than one drug to keep the bronchial tubes dilated. For this reason, we must now explore a second class of drugs that may be used to produce continuous bronchodilation. You must understand that often we mix classes of drugs although, ideally, we should try one class before we proceed to a second or even mix them.

The second group of medicines which produce continuous bronchodilation are the *methyl xanthines*. Many physicians believe they should be the first drug that an asthmatic tries for continuous dilation.

I want to emphasize this concept of twenty-four-hour bronchodilation. When you need it, you should take the medicine every four to six hours or otherwise you may not accomplish the desired effect.

All too often asthmatics delay taking drugs until they feel "bad enough," because they interpret "bad enough" as meaning needing it. These are the ostriches I referred to earlier. What they are doing is aggravating their problem. When such delays occur and the bronchoconstriction starts, it is more difficult to reverse the process. Delay in taking medicine results in variations rather than stable blood levels of the bronchodilators. A stable blood level of bronchodilators is more likely to prevent constriction from recurring.

We know, for example, that giving a bronchodilator *before exertion*, and especially when exposed to irritants or pollution, makes it much easier for the asthmatic than waiting for bronchospasm to start. When one gets a cold, a good routine is to be sure to use medication for bronchodilation *before* any spasm starts.

The problem of remembering to take medicine when one is feeling fairly good needs to be overcome in order to achieve maximum benefit from these drugs and ensure twenty-four-hour dilation. When dealing with the xanthines, keep in mind that there are short-acting and long-acting preparations. Since xanthines are mixed frequently with ephedrine compounds, one may be able to take the long-acting ones less frequently when asthma is mild. When asthma is more severe, however, short-acting medications may be required three, four, or more times a day. The best rule is to start taking the xanthine preparation at the earliest awareness of wheezing or chest tightness. Medication should be continued at the interval prescribed by your doctor throughout the day and for an arbitrary period of time, such as three or four days beyond the period when all feeling of wheezing has stopped. The reason for this is that a small degree of bronchial constriction will always be present even after all sounds or feelings of wheezing or tightness have disappeared, and when such constriction persists you are at a greater risk for further wheezing episodes.

The need for drugs, the period over which they should be taken, and the frequency, will vary with each asthmatic and may depend upon side-effects (Table 6, page 109). You will want to discuss this with your doctor. He may suggest you begin with a xanthine or an adrenalin-like compound. I prefer to begin with the xanthines. If this works, then the patient learns to use the medication on a regular basis when required. If the results are incomplete, one can add an adrenalin-like compound to the xanthine or try an adrenalin-like compound alone. Your doctor must make that decision with you, and the answer will depend very much upon his examination. Your understanding of how to take the medications, however, is the key to success.

Up to this point, I have not mentioned a number of the newer adrenergic drugs, which have essentially the same effect and were developed recently because they were thought to eliminate some of the unwanted side-effects on the heart. You should know, however, that they are not perfect. While they produce strong bronchodilation and their effect may last longer, they are not completely free of cardiac or nervous system stimulation.

The generic names of such medications are isoetharine (Bronkosol), salbutamol (Ventolin), protokylol (Ventaire), terbutaline (Brethine), (Bricanyl), and metaproterenol (Alupent) (Metaprel). Isoproterenol (Isuprel) has been known for a long time. It can also be used orally, but does produce unwanted side-effects. The point is that, if your doctor has prescribed one of these medications, you must ask him whether it is to be taken on a continuous basis. If so, understand that the drug falls into the continuous bronchodilation category. (See Table 7.)

To summarize:

1. A continuous program to achieve twenty-four-hour bronchodilation is essential for all those who have spasm on a daily or intermittent basis. It is not required during periods when you are asthma-free.

2. After all symptoms have subsided, it is advisable to treat for an additional three to four days to be sure that no residual bronchospasm exists.

3. The methyl-xanthine group is the most desirable group of drugs with which to begin such a program. They have the least side-effects.

TABLE 7. Oral Medications for Continuous Bronchodilation

Xanthine-containing Compounds	*Adrenalin-like Drugs*
Aerolate	**WITH EPHEDRINE**
Airet	Ascato Liquid*(OTC)
Amilixir*	Ectasule*
Aminodur	Ectasule minus
Aminophyllin	Rynatuss*
Amodrine*(OTC)	Slo-Fedrin
Asbron*	Wesmatic*
Brondecon*	
Bronkodyl	**WITHOUT EPHEDRINE**
Brophylline	Alupent
Choledyl	Brethine
Circair	Bricanyl
Dilor	Bronkosol
Dyphyllin	Isuprel
Elixophyllin	Metaprel
Emphaseem	Ventaire
G-Bron*	Ventolin
Hylate*	
Lanophyllin	**EPHEDRINE MIXED WITH XANTHINE**
Lixaminol	Asmac*(OTC)
Lufyllin	Asmasan*(OTC)
Neothylline	Asmaset*(OTC)
Neulin	Asmavert*(OTC)
Optiphyllin	Asminyl Tablets* (OTC)
Quibron*	Asno*(OTC)
Somophyllin	Asthmacon*(OTC)
Synophylate	Asthmadan*(OTC)
Tega-bron Elixir (OTC)	Asthmador (OTC)
Theobid	Asthmaid (OTC)
Theodide*(OTC)	Asthmanefrin (OTC)
Theodur	Azma-Aid Tablets (OTC)
Theofort	Azmar Tablets (OTC)
Theoguala (OTC)	Breatheasy*(OTC)
Theokin* (OTC)	Bronchotab* (OTC)
Theolair	Broncobid
Theolaphen*(OTC)	Brondecon
Theolix (OTC)	Bronitin (OTC)

TABLE 7. Continued

Xanthine-containing Compounds	Adrenalin-like Drugs
Theonar	Bronkolixir*(OTC)
Theo-organidin	Ephenyllin (OTC)
Theophyl	For-az-ma (OTC)
TSG-K1*	Neoasmasan*(OTC)
	Quadrinal*
	Sedral Tablets*(OTC)
	Tedral*(OTC)
	Thalfedrin*(OTC)
	Theodrine (OTC)
	Theofel*(OTC)
	Theophenedrine*(OTC)
	Verequad*(OTC)

*Contains a sedative, antihistamine, or other component.

OTC—Over-the-counter preparations sometimes differ from prescription items by having smaller doses of the medication. The term signifies that the medication can be purchased at the pharmacy without a doctor's prescription.

Note: A number of compounds contain pseudoephedrine or phenylephrine. They are normally used as cold tablets. Their bronchodilating effect is so weak that they are not included in this chart.

4. Ephedrine is a very commonly used drug, often mixed with the xanthines, but may be less desirable because of the frequency of the side-effects. Newer medications belonging to the adrenalin-like class and called beta-adrenergic drugs are becoming increasingly desirable.

5. Such newer drugs may be combined with the xanthines when required. The prophylactic use of such medicines, as at the onset of a cold or before exercise, is a valuable addition to an asthmatic's routine. List the medicines in this category under the "continuous" heading of your treatment program.

THE ACUTE ATTACK

In order to discuss an acute attack, it is first necessary to define it. Simply stated, any worsening of breathing which occurs within a relatively short period of time and does not respond to any of the usual continuous medication should be treated as an acute attack. Even when taking continuous medication, the asthmatic experiences times when bronchospasm increases and he feels more short of breath than he should. It is at this point that additional remedies may be required. The most commonly used and probably the most efficacious are the aerosol group of drugs. I want to emphasize, however, that the aerosols should be used only after one has been committed to a program designed to maintain twenty-four-hour control. The aerosols should not be used as a single, primary source of treatment. Before discussing the different types of aerosols and other possible treatments, make a second column on your treatment program worksheet and label this column: "Acute Attack."

Aerosols. There are four different kinds of aerosolization. The first kind, formerly used almost exclusively, has a hand nebulizer with a bulb at one end which you squeeze as you inhale. Two other types require much more equipment. These are the compressor-powered nebulizer and the IPPB devices. IPPB stands for intermittent positive pressure breathing. Both of these devices should be used only under your physician's guidance. Should there be a reason for using them, such as a fair amount of emphysema, then you should have special instruction.

Most asthmatics will use a Freon propellant which works like the spray cans that are currently on the market. When asthmatics use the aerosols too often, it is usually because of mistakes that are made frequently with Freon-propelled equipment. It is important to outline these errors. First, some asthmatics exhale rather than inhale as they squirt the dose. Others deliver the aerosol into the room instead of the mouth. Still others take a deep breath and *then* squirt the propellant, assuming that, because their lungs are filled as much as possible, the propellant will float down into the bronchial tubes while the breath is held. And, lastly, people often take too shallow an inspiration and follow that by exhaling immediately. This process simply blows the propellant out into the upper passages where it is frequently swallowed.

Most experts recommend the following:

1. An asthmatic should exhale comfortably so that the air in his lungs has reached the lowest comfortable level.

2. The nebulizer should be placed loosely in the mouth and inspiration should begin slowly rather than rapidly. It is important to understand that rapid expansion of the lungs, or a forced deep breath, does not produce as much expansion as a slow inspiration. The slower the inspiration, the greater the area over which the nebulized material is distributed. In the accompanying diagram (Figure 9), you will note that slow inspiration promotes distribution of the medication to areas where the airways are narrowed, while more rapid deep breathing results in accumulation of the medication in the larger airways where it is less needed.

3. The asthmatic should take two or three puffs, or squirts, of the medication during the single inspiration. This stimulates continuous flow of the drug.

4. After reaching maximum inhalation, the asthmatic should hold the breath and count to five slowly, so that the medication can be deposited on the surface of the airways before exhalation is begun.

It really is not complicated. Rather, it is a matter of learning how to do it properly. I would like to emphasize, however, that the above description should be considered *one treatment*. It is not to be repeated for a second or third time. Two or three squirts are the absolute maximum to be used in a treatment, and three or four treatments per day probably is the most that one should use the nebulizer unless required during the sleeping hours. A good rule to follow is that if you need a nebulizer more than every four hours to gain relief, you require medical advice.

As to whether or not one nebulizer is better than another, there is no special answer. There are a large number available containing adrenalin or adrenalin-like medication and some of the newer drugs. Table 8 contains a list of aerosols most commonly used. Discuss the different kinds with your physician and select that one that produces the most benefit and the least side-effects for you.

Incidentally, I must point out that the routine use of aerosols, or nebulizers, is controversial. There are some experts who strongly feel that, especially in children, they should *never* be prescribed. They argue that the nebulizers are overused, cause dependence, invite high risks of overdose, even perpetuate attacks, and produce

**THE BENEFITS OF SLOW INSPIRATION AND BREATH
HOLDING DURING NEBULIZATION**

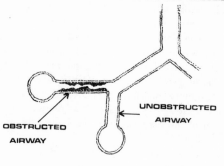

**OBSTRUCTED
AIRWAY**

**UNOBSTRUCTED
AIRWAY**

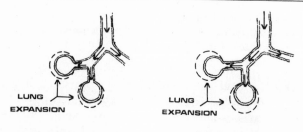

**LUNG
EXPANSION**

RAPID INSPIRATION

**LUNG
EXPANSION**

SLOW INSPIRATION

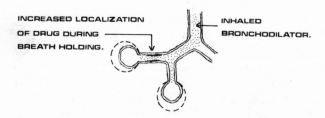

**INCREASED LOCALIZATION
OF DRUG DURING
BREATH HOLDING.**

**INHALED
BRONCHODILATOR.**

FIGURE 9.
Lung expansion is increased during slow inspiration and more bronchodilator drug reaches obstructed channels during breath holding.

TABLE 8. Pressurized Bronchodilation Aerosols

Generic Drug	Brand Name	Comments
Epinephrine	Asthma Meter Asthmanephrin (OTC) Asthmatan Mist (OTC) Breatheasy (OTC) Bronchaid Mist (OTC) Medihaler-Epi Metanephrine microNEPHRIN Primatene Mist (OTC) Vapomist (OTC) Vaponephrine	Controversial for acute attack. Some feel not appropriate for asthma, particularly not for children.
Isoetharine	Bronkometer	Controversial; new.
Isoproterenol	Duo-Medihaler Isuprel Kapo-N-Iso Medihaler ISO Mistometer Nor-isodrine Zuf-Iso	Controversial because of certain effects. Many feel these should not be used at all.
Metaproterenol	Alupent Metaprel	Controversial; new.
Salbutamol	Albuterol Ventolin	Not available in U.S.
Terbutaline	Brethine Bricanyl	Not available in U.S. as spray.

risks of fatality. For these reasons, before you list aerosols as a method of treatment for acute attack, be certain your doctor has agreed that they are indicated for you. I don't object to the proper use of nebulizers providing the frequency of use is restricted.

It is important to keep in mind that proper use of an aerosol means that the medication reaches the finest bronchial tubes, or bronchioles. This is essential for effective drug action. When the medication does not reach these levels, maximum response is prevented. There are three reasons why the spray may not reach the right areas. The first reason is improper breathing. Secondly, the particle size of the medication may be too large to enter the smallest airways. Finally, the degree of bronchoconstriction and mucus formation may be so great that penetration of the aerosol is prevented.

Not infrequently one sees asthmatics using the aerosols excessively. If an aerosol has been used properly, there should be sufficient relief so that there is no need for too frequent use. Of course, if the degree of bronchospasm is refractory, other methods of treatment may be required. Keep in mind the rule: Restrict usage to no more than three or four times a day.

Other Drugs for Acute Attack. During an acute attack, a stronger medication may be required because a state of "resistance," or reduced responsiveness to oral medications or aerosols, has occurred. Injections of adrenalin and xanthines are often given by doctors in such instances. The common routine in an emergency room, after taking the patient's blood pressure, is to administer an adrenalin injection because, by the time a patient has come there, he has tried most everything else. If adrenalin does not work after three injections twenty minutes apart, the next most common step is an intravenous injection of aminophyllin, a xanthine compound.

When an asthmatic develops an acute attack at home, another xanthine may be a theophyllin suppository or enema. (See Samples 1 and 3.) If you are an asthmatic who has needed to go to an emergency room, or to call a physician in the middle of the night, ask your physician whether or not you should store some suppositories to use on occasions when your asthma is "acute." Suppositories may afford you additional relief to avoid the need of an adrenalin injection.

On the other hand, an adrenalin injection may be essential for you.

The Question of Adrenalin Injections. Is it possible to give yourself an injection of adrenalin? If patients can readily learn to give themselves insulin for diabetes, why can't you be taught to inject yourself with adrenalin or epinephrine when you need it?

Well, first, before you learn *how* to give it, you need to learn *when* and *if* it should be given. To begin with, an injection is given when everything else has failed. Candidates for adrenalin injections are those who have had emergency room experience or have had to call a physician during the night because everything has been tried and nothing has worked.

I am not worried about recommending adrenalin for the "acute attack," because no one can get the medication without a prescription. Your doctor must outline for you the specific reasons for using it in your case, as well as when and under what conditions.

Thus, the first thing you must do in order to give yourself an adrenalin injection is to obtain a prescription from your physician. Should enough people want and be able to give their own adrenalin injections, I suspect that, in the near future, the pharmaceutical houses will prepare disposable syringes already loaded with the proper dose so that you can purchase everything you need in a single unit. Then you will simply have to wipe the area with an alcohol-impregnated swab and plop the needle under the skin.

At this time, however, preloaded syringes are not available. So in order to give an injection, you must learn how to take the medication from a vial into the syringe, how much to take up, and how to give the injection. Those three steps are essential. When your physician writes your prescription for adrenalin, he must also write a prescription for syringes and needles that you will need because, in most states, a doctor's order is necessary for both.

Adrenalin, or epinephrine, usually comes in a 10 cc vial in a 1:1000 strength. Ten cc's are about two teaspoonsful. An injection requires only a tiny amount—less than 1 cc. Since the adrenalin is tightly packaged, as you draw liquid out of the vial, you begin to create a vacuum. Therefore, it is necessary to put a little air into the bottle every time you prepare an injection. It is important to remember that, during the entire procedure, you are going to maintain a sterile technique. At no time will you touch the inside of the syringe, the needle, or the liquid with any object except the sterile needle tip. If you touch the needle, nothing is sterile any longer. Never place a used, or dirty, needle into the vial. That would contaminate the contents and make the medication unusable.

While this may sound complicated, it really isn't. Once you've gotten the knack of it, it's a simple procedure. If the concept worries you, just remember diabetics throughout the country give themselves injections every day. It's not difficult to learn, although it will be necessary to have your physician check you out after you have bought the equipment. The following steps summarize the procedure for giving an adrenalin injection:

1. Take your sterile syringe and draw about 0.5 cc of air into the barrel of the syringe. (I recommend that you use syringes which can be discarded after each injection. Use a 1 cc syringe of the tuberculin-type, with a No. 25 or No. 26 needle attached. These are the smallest-size needles and are used also for hypodermic injections.)

2. Wipe the top of the vial of adrenalin with a pledget of cotton soaked in rubbing alcohol. (You can use absorbent cotton on which you pour some rubbing alcohol, or you can buy disposable swabs, packaged in foil, which are impregnated with isopropyl alcohol, and are designed for this purpose.) This sterilizes the top of the vial. After a moment or two, when the alcohol on the top of the vial has dried, insert the sterile needle of the disposable syringe into the center of the vial and inject the air from the syringe.

3. Turn the vial upside down so that the tip of the needle lies underneath the adrenalin in the vial. (If the needle lies above the fluid, you would withdraw only air when you pull back the plunger on the syringe.) Withdraw 0.2 cc of adrenalin. Quickly remove the needle from the vial.

4. Prepare the arm or thigh for the injection by rubbing the area with the same pledget (or swab) of alcohol-saturated cotton.

5. Hold the syringe upright (needle pointing up) and carefully push up on the plunger until the adrenalin reaches the top end of the syringe, pushing out all the air. You are sure the air is out when a drop or two of adrenalin emerges from the upheld needle.

6. Quickly insert the needle, as if it were a dart, into the area of the arm or leg that you've wiped with the alcohol swab. (When this is done quickly, you'll be surprised how painless it is. Slow injections are difficult from a psychological point of view and also afford more time to feel the prick.)

7. Suck back on the contents by pulling the plunger back. This is to make sure no blood comes back through the needle. (It would be unlikely; but, if you were to aspirate some blood, you should withdraw the needle and inject at another site within the alcohol-wiped area.) When you see that there is no blood, quickly push down on the plunger and empty the contents of the syringe into the arm or leg.

Although I have indicated that many diabetics give themselves insulin, you must not assume that many asthmatics give themselves adrenalin injections. In fact, it is far from commonplace. Before you should consider learning to give an injection, first determine whether or not it is necessary.

Review the following:

1. Frequent need to call your physician for adrenalin injections, or
2. Frequent need to use a hospital emergency room, and
3. Rapid relief from adrenalin injections.

If your experiences include these, then it might be practical to learn how and when to give yourself injections. Discuss this with your doctor. What I'm suggesting is that your own experience will become the indication as to whether or when an injection is needed.

Now, under the second heading of your treatment program worksheet, list the medications you will use for an acute attack. Begin with an aerosol if you are currently using one. If you know it to be inadequate, you will need to ask your physician for alternatives. List those which he considers appropriate for you, and prescribes.

OTHER DRUGS

In addition to the medications used for continuous bronchodilation and for the "acute attack," there are three classes of drugs that should be considered for listing under a third column, which you shall label as "Other." Each of these three classes has different actions and each may be indicated for different reasons. It will be rare, though possible, that some asthmatics will require all three.

The first class is the antibiotics. The second class is the cortisone group. The third class is the newer medication called cromolyn sodium.

Each of these drugs carries a different brand name. If you are not sure if a medication prescribed for you falls within one of these classes, ask your physician or your pharmacist.

Earlier I mentioned that antihistamines could be listed here. If you do list them in the "other" category, then remember that they represent a fourth class. List them under "other," however, if you use them only intermittently.

Antibiotics. Because antibiotics are used for treatment of infections, many people believe that using one will prevent an infection. A patient once asked me why one shouldn't use antibiotics continuously for asthma.

"I have a neighbor who takes them all the time for acne," she said. "Shouldn't they be a good thing for an asthmatic?"

The answer is no.

If you took such a drug regularly, it would be like using a cannon to kill a fly. Of course, a fly can be terribly annoying, but every time you shot the cannon you could be knocking holes in a lot of other things unnecessarily. For the asthmatic, the goal is to have things available to be used if needed, not to be loaded down with all kinds of pills and sprays. The example of acne is a good one. Acne is a skin condition in adolescents. One acne type develops frequent infections due, usually, to a staphylococcus germ. This type of acne patient has reddened, angry-looking pimples that begin to resemble boils. Sometimes they have to be lanced. The dermatologists know that tetracycline (an antibiotic) frequently neutralizes the staph infection and that a very small dose, often just one capsule a day, can control the infection.

If an asthmatic's bronchial tubes get to look like the skin of an acne patient, the doctor must prescribe an antibiotic, and must determine the length of time the asthmatic needs to take it. There are some people, usually those with a long-standing chronic bronchitis and other lung complications, who may benefit from long-term antibiotics. What it comes down to is whether or not an infection is present and what will be required to cure it.

To test for an infection, your doctor may request a "culture" of the sputum. When the sputum is clear, an infection is not usually present, but when the sputum becomes yellow or green the possibility does exist. A culture determines if a germ is present and helps the doctor decide which antibiotic to use.

To summarize: Like most of the adolescents with acne, the majority of asthmatics do *not* need an antibiotic when they have an asthma attack. But if an infection is present in the body, as in acute or chronic bronchitis, then your doctor may consider using an antibiotic. But because antibiotics are cannons and they can have side-effects, they must be used wisely.

Cortisone or Steroid Drugs. The cortisone compounds, or steroids, as they often are called, are another class of medications which may be even bigger cannons. As a matter of fact, a cannon is a bad analogy. The steroids don't go off with a bang. Instead, they often make you feel better. They are like an invisible ray because their side-effects are very subtle and often the asthmatic is unaware of what can be happening when he takes steroids.

Earlier, we considered how these drugs may work. Now I want to introduce three terms which should help you whenever you may need to take a medicine: indication, contraindication, and side-effects.

Indication means: "What are the reasons to take a medicine?" Contraindication means just the opposite: "What are the reasons that could prohibit using a medicine?" Side-effects are the possible things that the medicine can do besides curing the condition.

In every instance, the benefits, or the indications, must outweigh the contraindications and the risk of the side-effects. Cortisone-like drugs are a good example of the need for this kind of reasoning. If you look at the list of possible side-effects (Table 9), you will see that stomach ulcer, or high blood pressure, are noted. This doesn't mean that every patient will get either or both, but the doctor must consider the possibility. If there is a history of a previous ulcer or the presence of high blood pressure, then the doctor must consider the risk of possible recurrence. The history of an ulcer, or the presence

TABLE 9. Possible Long-Term Side-Effects of Steroid Therapy

Hormone Changes	*Other Medical Effects*
Loss of your own adrenal gland function, especially under stress	High blood pressure
	Peptic ulcer
Rounding of the face	Loss of bone calcium
Weight gain	Behavior changes
Elevated blood sugar or diabetes	Acne
Excessive hair growth on face	Salt and water retention
	Increased liability to infection

These effects depend upon length of steroid intake, dose, and individual variations.

of high blood pressure, then become a *relative* contraindication to the medication. I say "relative" because, under certain conditions, the doctor may try a steroid in the hope that the particular patient won't develop those side-effects. In fact, he might even give ulcer medication, or pills for high blood pressure, simultaneously, to prevent such possible side-effects.

The important thing about steroids is that they are saved for those individuals who do not respond to anything else. In fact, at times, they are life-saving. They neutralize the asthma so well that the asthmatic is reluctant to stop them. On the other hand, one of the safe things about steroids is the fact that side-effects occur only after they have been used for a considerable period. It is rare to have a problem in less than a few weeks. For this reason, they frequently are used when hospitalization is required for very severe attacks.

Even more important, if the asthma is bad enough, there may be no other choice. Just make sure your physician regulates the amount you take. The best plan, one most doctors use, is to start with a large dose, and then rapidly taper the dose to the least amount that can be comfortably tolerated. Prednisone and prednisolone are the two most commonly used steroids. (These are generic, not brand names and so they are the least expensive.) Generally, doctors try to keep the dose below three tablets daily, especially if one is required to take them for long periods. One trick that sometimes is used is to give the medication every second day. Alternate doses of 20 mg. of prednisone are well tolerated by some adult asthmatics.

To sum up, the strategy is to stop a severe attack as quickly as possible to prevent a worsening or self-perpetuating attack, and then reduce the dose and eliminate the drug as soon as a wheeze-free status is achieved.

The purpose of the table showing side-effects is to create a healthy respect for the cortisone-like compounds. But more than that, I would like to introduce a concept of treatment that patients rarely understand. The concept is that of seduction. People want to get better. Often they don't care *how* as long as they see results occurring quickly. Doctors, too, like to satisfy their patients. Both can be *seduced* into treatments that work, but which can only cause trouble in the long run. For example, the concomitant use of a round-the-clock nebulizer and long-term use of steroids should be condemned. I can't emphasize enough that just because something works well doesn't mean that you should use it.

On the other hand, we need an arsenal of agents to attack asthma. The more things we have available, the more we can select. I use steroids when bronchodilation fails, but I use it for short periods and quickly reduce the dose. In some cases, it must be used for longer periods under careful medical control. When proper precautions are taken, risks become minimal.

Aerosol steroids have been used in Europe and are now on the market in this country. The newer ones are minimally absorbable. By that I mean that they don't get out of the lungs into the body, so that the list of side-effects is not applicable (Table 10).

We haven't found the ideal medication yet. The steroid spray seems to be extremely helpful for asthmatics. But like everything else, it may have side-effects too. Its greatest benefit, though, may be to enable elimination of use of oral steroids or significantly reduce the dosage. But the steroid aerosol is new. We haven't used it enough to know the long-term effects. We do know that it can be slightly irritating and that a monilial, or yeast, infection of the bronchial tubes has been reported. It requires a prescription, so your physician must make the decision as to whether or not you can use it.

When a physician describes potential dangers to a patient, there

TABLE 10. Other Aerosols

Generic Drug	Brand Name	Comments
STEROID AEROSOLS		
Beclomethasone	Becotide Vanceril	Used for severe asthma only with remarkable benefit. Has local effect with minimum absorption into the general system. Reduces need for oral cortisone
Triamcinolone	Beclomet	Absorbed into general circulation; should be used rarely, if ever
MEDIATOR INHIBITOR		
Cromolyn Sodium	Aarane Intal	Acts gradually over a period of time by inhibiting mediators of allergy. The aerosol has a propeller-like gadget so that proper use is essential.

is always a tendency to alarm the person. Nothing is one hundred percent safe—not even your automobile. But if you drive carefully, carry out preventive maintenance when indicated, and watch out for the "crazies" on the road, you can get a lot of mileage under your belt. Different from an automobile driver, the asthmatic has a physician as an advisor on whom he can call—something like having a "co-pilot" on a long trip.

Cromolyn Sodium. The third drug under "other" is cromolyn sodium. Cromolyn sodium is relatively safe. It is rather expensive, can be irritating, is a bit troublesome to use, but only rarely is associated with a serious sensitivity (Table 10).

"It's also like my car when the battery is dead," a patient remarked recently. "Nothing happens when you use it."

In a way, she was right. It does not cause bronchodilation. It probably works by inhibiting the effect of those agents which mediate or cause an allergic cellular response. You see no immediate results, and you must use it daily—several times a day—with a special gadget containing a tiny propeller. You take a capsule, place it in a tiny receptacle in the inhaler, puncture it with a tiny pin that operates by sliding a "sleeve" on the inhaler, and then inhale the powder contained in the capsule into the lungs. It is different from a nebulizer because a sucking breath is required to pull the powder from the capsule into the lungs. Many asthmatics get the powder only as far back as the throat instead of the lungs, and neutralization of the substances which produce bronchodilation begins to develop gradually.

Despite these drawbacks, results may be dramatic for some. Indications are for the allergic asthmatic who does not have twenty-four-hour bronchodilation and has, or requires, additional, or more continuing, steroid therapy. It should be used three to four times daily for at least a month before being abandoned as "ineffective." Within a thirty-day period, it can be found to be very helpful indeed. What one usually notes in those who obtain benefit is a decreasing need for other medications. In those who respond, dosage sometimes can be reduced to two or three times a day, but even then there can be "breakthrough" attacks requiring regular forms of treatment.

SAMPLE 1. My Treatment Program

Continuous Bronchodilation
1. Choledyl every four hours
2. Marax every six hours

Acute Attack
1. Bricanyl
2. Aminophyllin
   suppositories

Other
1. Teldrin spansules*
2. Aristocort
3. Aarane 3 times a day

*Long-acting antihistamine

Note: Since dosages vary for adults and children, and from asthmatic to asthmatic, they are not listed here.

SAMPLE 2. My Treatment Program

Continuous Bronchodilation
1. Elixophyllin every six hours
2. Ephedrine 3 times a day
3. Chlor-Trimeton, long-acting, at bedtime

Acute Attack
1. Alupent

Other
   None

I suggest that cromolyn sodium be placed in the "other" column rather than the "continuous" group because it doesn't produce twenty-four-hour bronchodilation and the "continuous" group of drugs really refers to that effect. Cromolyn sodium has a longer-term, anti-allergic effect.

At this point, review your treatment program worksheets. The samples on pages 157–158 show three examples of moderate and moderately severe asthmatic treatment plans. Complete your own plan, using what you take now after consulting with your doctor and arranging for your best program. Do you feel it is adequate and that you understand where each of your medications belongs? Check

SAMPLE 3. My Treatment Program

Continuous Bronchodilation
1. Quibron 4 times a day
2. Tedral S.A. in A.M.

Acute Attack
1. Theophyllin enema
2. Medihaler-epi
3. Adrenalin injections

Other
1. Ampicillin*

*Antibiotic

with the charts which show the different classes of medications. If necessary, reread sections of this chapter. You should have enough information to classify your medications.

On the other hand, you may realize that there are additional things that you might be able to do for yourself. On your worksheet, list questions that occur to you and be sure to raise them on your next visit with your doctor. Your treatment program is the final section of your Personal Asthma Contract, and the information from your worksheet should now be added. You should then put at the very bottom "I commit myself to controlling my asthma" and sign your name.

This section is the only one which needs continuing review. Your medication needs may change; but even more important, new drugs will continue to become available. You now know what questions to ask about your pills and liquids and sprays and suppositories. When you have completed this final portion of your contract, your form should be similar to that of the sample contract for John Jones (pages 160–161).

"What do I do for *continuous bronchodilation* and for an *acute attack?*"

"What other things are available?"

"What are the indications, contraindications, and side-effects?"

"Are my needs greater than the risks?"

These are the questions you must answer. Now that you have completed your education, you are an informed asthmatic. You can treat yourself wisely. Your doctor is your expert consultant. The two of you, working together, will prove that breathing easy can be attained.

(SAMPLE)

MY PERSONAL ASTHMA CONTRACT

Name: John Jones   Date: January 1, 19—

Goal I. Gain Understanding of Asthma   Date Completed
   1) General Knowledge   Jan. 1
   2) Specific Knowledge About Myself   Jan. 3
      a) My General Medical History
      b) My Emotional History
      c) My Allergic History
   3) My Asthma Pattern:
      PERENNIAL, MIXED ASTHMA   Jan. 5
   4) My Medications History for: Jan. 6
      a) Asthmatic Attack
        PRIMATENE MIST
        TEDRAL
      b) Allergy
        CHLOR-TRIMETON
      c) Infection
        PENICILLIN
      d) Other
   5) Trigger Factors: Jan. 8
      a) General
        DAMPNESS
        SMOKE
        CIGARETTES
        COLD WEATHER
        FISH ODORS
      b) Emotional
        ANGER WITH BOSS (UNEXPRESSED)
      c) Allergic
        RAGWEED
        GRASSES
        FISH?
      d) Other
Goal II. Develop Prevention Program
   1) Physician Consultation: Jan. 10

a) "Histories" Review	Jan. 10
b) Additional Examinations	
Physical examination	Jan. 10
Special breathing tests	none
Blood tests	none
X-rays	none
EKG	none
Allergy studies	years ago
2) Allergy Prevention:	
a) Create dust-free environment	Jan. 13
b) Plan an elimination diet	not indicated
c) Desensitization	not indicated
3) Stop Smoking	not indicated
4) Establish Procedure for:	
a) Air Pollution or Inclement Weather	Jan. 10
b) Upper Respiratory Infection	Jan. 10
5) Establish Breathing and General Exercise Program	Jan. 17
Goal III. Develop Treatment Program	Jan. 20

1) Continuous Bronchodilation

ELIXOPHYLLIN

CHLOR-TRIMETON

BRETHINE

2) Acute Attack

MEDIHALER

3) Other

CROMOLYN SODIUM

ERYTHROMYCIN WHEN PRESCRIBED

I commit myself to controlling my asthma.

Signature _____

Date Jan. 20, 19--

13

Controlling Your Asthma

It was a quiet Sunday afternoon. It had stopped raining and the smell of spring was in the air. I had just finished reviewing a complicated article on a new class of cellular enzymes, called prostaglandins, which may affect the balance of chemical substances in the lungs of an asthmatic. Suddenly I realized that the day that was nice for me could be miserable for an allergic asthmatic: the slight dampness, the spring pollens. What a perfect setting for an attack!

Medical attempts to control asthma are increasingly effective, but the settings which induce the production of these unfavorable lung substances that cause bronchial constriction are increasing. Unless environmentalists can force society to keep fresh air fresh, newer medical controls will continue to be necessary.

Medical research benefits the asthmatic. During the 1960s, great strides were made in distinguishing the different kinds of asthmatics. Understanding the chemical substances which interrelate and cause bronchoconstriction has been another major, and more recent, advance. Even now, medical science is approaching the point of applying new concepts to the development of new drugs.

The practicality of research is based upon the expectation that continued search will materially benefit patients and upon the recognition of the increasing prevalence of asthma. Roughly estimated, there are now 10 asthmatics for every 1,000 people (or one percent of the population), although the rate for children under 16 is between five and fifteen percent, or 50 to 150 asthmatics per 1,000 children.

The known and accepted facts about asthma continue to be updated. Because it is among the leading causes of time lost from school and work, it is a significant reason for continued doctor-patient contacts. And because of these contacts, opportunities continue to occur for each asthmatic to become knowledgeable about his own asthma, to learn new ways and modes of treatment as they develop, and to be as totally proficient in self-care as possible.

The need for you to be proficient is the basis for this book. The guidelines which now you should have worked out through your contract can remain the basis of your asthma treatment unless a disease process changes your condition. Because such an instance is rare, many, or perhaps even most, of the decisions that will have to be made for your best possible breathing may be made by you. Lisa is an example of an asthmatic who has become self-proficient.

Lisa is a young photographer for a major television network. She has had asthma since her childhood. She has a series of known allergies, but her asthmatic episodes probably occurred more frequently after respiratory infections than after exposure to allergens, although both were important.

Over the years, Lisa has learned increasingly how to combat her asthmatic episodes. One afternoon she called me, complaining that her asthma had worsened. She had just purchased a new rug and was concerned whether the attacks were an allergic response to the fibers of the new rug. During our discussion, she reminded herself that her recent attacks had begun prior to the time the rug was laid.

"It seems to me that I caught another cold about a month ago," she remarked. "My breathing has been rotten since then, but the rug could be a factor, couldn't it?"

"What kind of a rug is it? Is it wool or cotton?" I asked.

"Neither," she replied. "It's one of those synthetics—a polyester rug. But aren't allergic reactions to such materials uncommon?"

"Yes," I answered. "More usually an allergy would be related to dust that might accumulate in them."

"But the rug's new, so there's been no time for dust to accumulate," she said.

A few days later she came into my office with a sample of the rug.

"I'm quite sure my rug has nothing to do with my breathing problem," she said, "but I'd like you to check it out for me anyway. I've slept away from my apartment and remained as much as possible out of the room where the new rug is laid, but my asthma has continued. I'm coughing up yellowish-green mucus and my head feels terrible. I don't have any toothaches like the time when my sinuses were inflamed, but I suspect that I should get an antibiotic. A friend of mine gave me one of those Contac capsules to decongest my nose but I found it was too drying for my breathing. I think that if I continue on the Elixophyllin and Marax, take an antibiotic and an antihistamine, and get rid of this cough, I'll do well again."

"I think you're right," I said. "I agree with everything you've said. I don't know how many doctors would admit it, but I can't add anything except to write you an antibiotic prescription and review anything else you need. You really don't have need for me, do you?"

"Oh, yes, I do," she replied. "I need you to reassure me and advise me when I might be wrong. I know that asthmatic attacks are guesswork. Even though I know pretty much about myself and how I react, you are a great help."

Her response delighted me. I realized that Lisa had reached the basic level that I am trying to get people to achieve. In situations that are chronic and/or recurrent, each person learns his own lessons. He knows his own rules and what happens when he breaks them.

You too should now be at that level. Your doctor may be your lifeline to safety, but it is you who must now move in the right direction. Your doctor can only tell you which way. Hopefully, when new discoveries are pertinent, he will advise you about what could be helpful for you.

For example, the new steroid aerosol will be dramatic aid for a large number of asthmatics. Still it is *not* the proper treatment for many. New adrenalin and xanthine-like compounds with less and less side-effects, newer atropine-like, or special anti-allergic substances, or perhaps even enzymes or totally different chemical compounds may also appear and benefit large numbers of people. But there will always be those who require few if any medications. Remember, the psychological aspects of asthma cannot be ignored. Such avenues as meditation, or special relaxation programs, should be explored by some.

For many, the contract may provide a kind of "daily schedule," a list of rules or regulations. For you, perhaps, it will be less strict—more a group of reminders. If you review your contract from time to time, you may want to update your knowledge by asking your doctor for references on the latest concepts.

Below I have listed fifteen general guidelines as a final summary list. As you review them, you will notice that many of them are part of your Personal Asthma Contract. Add any to your contract that you think will provide additional emphasis. But incorporate only those things which you really need. Don't complicate your life with rules, unless rules make your life less complicated. Find time for the pleasures that come with breathing easy.

Summary List—Ways to Control My Asthma

1. Don't work or play beyond the point of fatigue. (Hard to do? Of course, but what is the best use of time? Don't work when you are knowingly overtired. It is much better to stop at the point of fatigue, rest, and pick up again at a later hour.)

2. Get adequate sleep—seven or eight hours a night.

3. Don't smoke.

4. Make your daily diet contain the six essential nutrients—protein, fat, carbohydrates, vitamins, minerals, and water.

5. Drink a minimum of eight glasses of water every day; drink more to stave off, or "break," an asthma attack.

6. Avoid all foods to which you are knowingly allergic.

7. Do breathing exercises, preferably in the morning and in the evening not long before sleep.

8. Spend fifteen to sixty minutes daily in other exercise—swimming, skating, bowling, dancing, calisthenics, walking, or other.

9. Endeavor to avoid environmental conditions that trigger your attacks—whether dust, fresh paint, smoke, gasoline fumes, gas, heat, or humidity. If you can't avoid them, reduce your activities to the

barest minimum while you are exposed to them. Consider prophylactic bronchodilators if an attack is expected.

10. Take medications prescribed for you regularly and
routinely—as your doctor ordered.

11. Carry a list of your medications in your billfold or purse.

12. Keep your Personal Asthma Contract posted where it's readily
visible to you and can be found by anyone helping you should you
have an acute attack.

13. Keep a diary so you'll be able to see that, *when you take
charge,* you can control your asthma and reduce or eliminate attacks.
(The diary will be reassuring to you and will be helpful to your doctor
should you have one of those decreasingly frequent attacks.)

14. Develop a meaningful hobby free of stress or undue physical
exertion, to help you take your mind from things you may have to
give up, such as smoking, being a wine expert, or playing tennis.
(Learning to play a wind instrument would help your breathing.)

15. Practice inviting serenity into your life—through any technique enjoyable to you.

And sign your contract with the conviction that *you* can control
your asthma, and breathe easy.

Appendix

DUST-FREE ENVIRONMENT

If the asthmatic is a mother or a housewife, hire someone to do the housecleaning. When that is not feasible, the asthmatic homemaker should wear a mask to lessen the amount of dust inhaled during the cleaning process.

Do not use insect sprays or other sprays. Avoid irritating paint, camphor, pine oils, and moth balls, and do not allow anyone to smoke in a dust-free bedroom.

Clean the bedroom once a week, more often if possible. Instead of a broom, use a cloth and mops moistened with water or, if you or another occupant of the dust-free room is not allergic to fumes, moisten the mop and dusting cloth with lightweight mineral oil. Avoid floor waxes and furniture polish.

Keep the closet doors and bedroom door closed at all times to avoid cooking and other irritating odors or dust from other parts of the home.

Vacuum the rest of the home at least once a week, including all over-stuffed furniture and draperies.

Eliminate venetian blinds. Use washable curtains or none.

An exhaust fan is recommended for the kitchen to remove cooking odors. If an allergy to gas fumes exists, it is sometimes necessary to substitute an electric cooking range.

To Create a Dust-free Bedroom

Floor should be hard wood, vinyl, or linoleum. If an area rug is used, it should be small, washable, and synthetic.

Remove *everything* from the room (furniture, bed, curtains, dresser). Empty the closets.

Wash room thoroughly with soap and water, including doors, baseboards—everything.

If the room contains an air conditioner, it should be cleaned and a new filter installed. The filter should be changed regularly.

Room Content

Use minimum amount of furniture. Cover mattress and box springs with an "allergen-proof" casing, not the usual plastic one. (See Resource List on page 183).

Avoid pillows stuffed with feathers, down, cotton linters, or kapok. Use a pillow made of foam rubber, urethane sponge, or synthetic fiber, but be aware that some may be sensitive to sponge rubber and if you use foam rubber, inspect it periodically. Be aware that molds sometimes grow in sponge rubber.

Use cotton, rayon, or synthetic fiber blankets, or wool, unless there is a wool sensitivity.

Use washable bedspreads. Avoid tufted and chenille ones.

Only keep clothing in closets currently being used. Do not store outer clothing or non-seasonal clothing, mementos, or other household articles in bedroom closets.

Ventilation

Avoid damp or excessively cold or humid air in the bedroom at night. Keep the windows closed, with the door open into an adjoining room which has an open window, or keep the windows open at the top no more than the width of a pencil, or, unless there is an adverse reaction, use an air conditioner.

If a radiator is used, it should be topped with a pan or tray of water. A humidifying device can be helpful to some asthmatics.

Other

If the home is old and there is a damp basement or dusty attic, give consideration to the existence of mold. If mold exists, have the attic and basement professionally sprayed. (See Resource List on page 183.)

BREATHING EXERCISES

Breathing is something most of us take completely for granted and never think about unless we get into trouble. Similarly, between attacks, most asthmatics don't think about breathing any more than non-asthmatics do. Westerners trained in certain Yoga teachings often practice breathing exercises. Houdini, the master magician and escape artist, was an expert in controlled breathing. For an asthmatic determined to bring his asthma under control so that he can breathe easy, and for mothers and fathers of asthmatics who want to give their children all help possible, breathing exercises should become a basic and important part of the asthma contract. You don't need to set a goal requiring the kind of control that Houdini practiced, but you might well put into your contract a clause specifying you will practice correct breathing at least twice a day—in the morning, before breakfast, and at night, before getting into bed—as well as at the first sign of impending attack to prevent asthma from coming on. Many asthmatics have found they can prevent their attacks simply by gentle breathing exercises.

If the asthmatic is short of breath or even wheezing slightly, a bronchodilator may make it feasible to perform the exercises with ease. Sometimes exercises do cause coughing at the end of an expiration, loosening the mucus in the bronchial tubes. Elimination of the mucus may further improve the breathing.

At first it may seem strange to do the exercises properly, particularly since it is common for the asthmatic's breathing to become increasingly shallow. This is a direct result of the fact that while the asthmatic can often get air into the lungs fairly easily during an attack, there is great difficulty in expelling the air. As a consequence, the lungs become overdistended, causing the diaphragm to flatten and be limited in its movement.

As the asthmatic uses the upper chest muscles more and more, breathing becomes increasingly shallow. If attacks last a long time or recur frequently, the lungs remain overdistended. The asthmatic then is constantly out of breath or starts to wheeze upon exertion.

There are informal breathing exercises, such as blowing up a balloon, and indirect breathing exercises, as practicing with certain musical instruments, such as a flute, clarinet, or trumpet. There is real evidence that regular practice with a wind instrument can be extremely beneficial. It's a way of getting in a lot of very beneficial breathing exercise while learning or developing a delightful skill as a hobby or profession.

Formal breathing exercises developed by research and medical groups, including the American Academy of Pediatrics and the British Asthma Research Council, are aimed at teaching how to breathe with the lower chest and abdominal muscles, including the diaphragm, rather than the upper chest and neck muscles.

Breathing Exercises

A.

1. Breathe in through the nose, gently, counting to yourself as you do so. Hold your hand on your abdomen and notice that, when you breathe with your diaphragm, your abdomen will extend during inspiration.

2. Breathe out through the mouth, counting to yourself for at least twice as long as you breathed in. Hold your hand on your upper abdomen and pull in the abdominal muscle during expiration.

Repeat three times.

B.

1. Lie on back on floor or firm mattress. Relax body. Rest hands on upper abdomen. Draw knees up into bent position. Breathe in gently, through the nose.

2. Breathe out slowly, through the mouth, gently sinking the chest and then upper abdomen until the abdomen is retracted at the end of a long, gentle expiration.

3. Relax upper abdomen. Breathe in gently through the nose. Do not raise chest.

4. Breathe out gently through the mouth as directed. Repeat eight to sixteen times. Rest one minute. Repeat.

C.

1. Sit in a straight-backed chair. Relax. Place palms of hands on each side of lower ribs.

2. Inhale gently through the nose.

3. Exhale slowly through the mouth, contracting upper part of thorax, then lower ribs, and then press palms against ribs to expel air from the bottom of the lungs.

4. Inhale while expanding upper abdomen and raising trunk slowly.
hands.

5. Repeat eight to sixteen times. Rest one minute. Repeat.

D.

1. Sit in a straight-backed chair. Relax arms at sides. Spread feet and knees apart.

2. Inhale gently through nostrils.

3. Exhale slowly through the mouth while dropping head forward and downward to knees. Retract abdominal muscles during latter part of forward bend.

4. Inhale while expanding upper abdomen and raising trunk slowly.

5. While remaining erect, exhale quickly, sinking chest and abdomen.

6. Inhale, expanding upper abdomen.

7. Repeat four to six times. Rest one minute. Repeat.

Between the different breathing exercises, practice the elbow exercise:

Elbow Exercise

1. Sit in straight-backed chair. Keep back straight, put fingers on shoulders, with elbows level with shoulders and lean forward slightly.

2. Rotate elbows in a circle.

3. Repeat four to eight times.

Once an asthmatic learns to exercise properly, some find they can prevent an attack simply by doing the breathing exercises. Once the asthmatic masters this, there is an automatic increase in confidence that asthma can be conquered.

Remember the basic goal is to learn how to use the diaphragm properly so as to move air in and out of the lungs with the least amount of work. Work is a good word here because, while for most people breathing is effortless, for the asthmatic, during an attack, breathing is work that uses up more oxygen than is taken in.

THE ELIMINATION DIET

Very few persons will take the time to test themselves for possible allergic reaction to such a comprehensive list of foods, inhalants, and contact allergens as is contained in Chapter 7. Where food allergies are suspected but not precisely identified, physicians often recommend that asthmatics go on an "elimination diet," eating foods known to be "safe" and causing no allergic reactions over a four to ten day period. After relief from allergic symptoms has been established for several days, individual foods are then added to the diet, one at a time, as a single meal taken between usual meals, such as at 11 A.M., 3 P.M., and 8 P.M. In starting this procedure, a food not normally causing allergic reactions is chosen, such as rice. The food is taken daily for five to seven days before trying another and the results carefully evaluated. If no allergic manifestation occurs, this food can then be added to the basic diet. If rice is the food chosen for the first test, white rice, brown rice, and puffed rice can be tested in rotation, but rice pudding cannot be included because that dish contains milk and eggs which are not part of the basic diet and are not recommended for testing until the patient has been on the "elimination diet" for a longer period.

A vegetable might be the second food chosen for the test. Response to individual vegetables usually can be adequately determined in a single test meal. This holds true of meats, fish, and fruits as well; but many foods, such as rice and wheat and eggs and milk and cheese, must be tested for several days since it has been found that, in some cases, adverse reactions do not occur at first. Of course, if an adverse reaction occurs with the first test meal, that product is not tested further, unless to check the certainty of the reaction and rule out a coincidence.

After the addition of vegetables, fruits, meats, poultry, fish, spices, and nuts may be added gradually. When dairy products are tested finally, start with pasteurized cow's milk and go on to cheeses, with separate meals for each cheese commonly eaten, such as American cheese, Swiss cheese, Cheddar cheese, and so forth.

Cereals then can be tested, again one at a time. Since many people are allergic to molds and because certain molds are common to all cereal grains, some people may not be able to eat any cereal without an adverse reaction.

After avoidance for two or three months of an allergen-producing food, it is sometimes possible to reintroduce safely a "favorite" food into the diet, even though there was an adverse reaction earlier.

Caution recommends that any food-sensitive person rotate allowed foods regularly, day after day. There is an additional benefit in rotating foods. The variety ensures a more adequate intake of all the nutrients needed to create and maintain a healthy internal environment.

Below is a list of "allowed foods," which should be eaten throughout the testing period except for the test meals. Of course, if a person suspects any of these "allowed" foods of causing adverse reactions, they too should be eliminated from the "basic diet," and tested at a later time, after allergic symptoms have subsided. The allergic person should eat nothing but allowed foods for a period of ten days to two weeks before starting to test any other food.

Foods Allowed

MEAT AND POULTRY
Bacon
Beef
Chicken
Lamb
Liver
Turkey
VEGETABLES
Artichoke
Asparagus
Beets
Carrots
Chard
Lettuce
Spinach
Squash
String beans
Tomato*
Zucchini
FRUITS
Apricots
Grapefruit
Lemon
Papaya
Peaches
Pears
Pineapple
Prunes
MISCELLANEOUS
Arrowroot
Baking powder (corn-free)

*Some asthmatics do not tolerate tomatoes well.

Baking soda
Cane or beat sugar
Cream of tartar
Gelatin—lemon, lime, or pineapple flavor, as well as plain
Lemon extract
Maple syrup
Salt—table, sea salt*
Sesame oil
Soy bean bread
Soy bean flour
Soy bean milk and butter
Soy bean oil
Tapioca
Vanilla extract
White vinegar

The following foods should be avoided completely during the testing period except for the individual food being tested after the ten-day or two-week allergen-free period.

Foods Not Allowed

DAIRY PRODUCTS
Butter
Cheese, except cottage and cream cheese
Milk, cream, ice cream
Oleomargarines
VEGETABLES
Beans, except string beans
Broccoli
Brussel sprouts
Cabbage
Cauliflower
Celery
Cucumber
Green peas
Green peppers
Lentils

*Some asthmatics find it necessary to eliminate table salt entirely.

Mustard
Onion
Parsley
Potato, sweet
Potato, white
Radish, horseradish
Turnips

FRUITS

Apples, raw
Avocado
Cantaloupe
Honeydew melon
Raisins
Strawberry
Watermelon

MISCELLANEOUS

Ale, beer
Carbonated drinks, including colas, ginger ale, etc.
Chocolate, cocoa
Coffee, unless freshly brewed by single filtration method and not boiled or reheated
Condiments or any highly spiced foods
Foods fried in vegetable oils such as cottonseed, soy, peanut, and corn
Nut butters
Nuts of any kind
Salad oils, including French dressing and mayonnaise prepared from vegetable oils
Tea—if boiled

Since some people have adverse reactions to the chlorine or fluorine in water, often mineral or store-bought spring water is recommended for drinking and cooking instead of water that comes from the faucet. Spring, mineral, or distilled water should therefore be given your strongest consideration.

It must be emphasized that each test meal is to be of a *single* food—raw, boiled, or baked—with nothing added other than *possibly* salt—sea or table salt.

A diary should be kept in which you record the times that test meals are eaten, the food that is eaten, and the reactions to the foods. It should include an account of all symptoms occurring during the night and upon arising in the morning. The diary also should include a listing of foods and snacks eaten throughout the day, and drinks consumed, as well as exposure to dust, chemical fumes, odors, pollens, molds, and pets.

Stress situations and feelings of anxiety and distress also should be recorded, as well as incidents creating happiness and pleasure.

THE WHEAT-FREE DIET

Wheat, milk, corn, and eggs are the leading offenders among allergen-producing foods. Thousands of varieties of wheat are grown, but sensitivity to one can mean sensitivity to all. While some people, after an extended period of abstinence, can reintroduce wheat into the diet safely, others can never eat it, or any food containing a wheat ingredient, without becoming symptomatic. Further, wheat can cause trouble not only as an ingestant but also as an inhalant.

The list of wheat-containing foods below is fairly comprehensive but it is by no means complete. There are many other products that also contain wheat. When a star * appears beside the product, that means that certain brands, or types, can be wheat-free. Read the labels and, if you are allergic to wheat, when dining out be sure to ask that foods be served plain, free of sauces or gravies.

Foods to Avoid

Alcoholic beverages containing grain neutral spirits (gin, whiskies)
Bread and rolls*
Breaded meat
Cakes
Canned soup
Chocolate
Cookies and crackers
Creamed soup unless thickened with egg, cornstarch, or arrowroot
Doughnuts
Gravies unless thickened with egg, cornstarch, or arrowroot
Ice cream cones
Macaroni and spaghetti*
Muffins, popovers, pretzels
Noodles

Pancakes and waffles
Pies
Wheat cereals—Wheatena, bran, cream of wheat, farina, shredded wheat, wheaties, puffed wheat
Wheat germ
Wieners

Foods Allowed

All fruits
All vegetables, raw or cooked
Corn bread
Corn, oat, or rice cereal
Cornstarch or rice pudding
Custards, junket
Fresh fish, meat, or poultry
Jello, fruit ice, or sherbet
Rice flour muffins or bread
Rye bread, if 100 percent rye†
Rye Krisp or Rye Kingwafers†

THE EGG-FREE DIET

While an allergy to eggs is not as common as to wheat, the egg-sensitive person can have a much more severe reaction simply by ingesting a product containing a minute amount of egg. Some of the products below carry a star * beside them, indicating that there are some store-bought brands and types that are egg-free, and of course you can make some of these foods at home using egg substitutes.

Foods to Avoid

Baking powder*
Bavarian cream

†Before using these products, test yourself to make sure that you are not allergic to rye as well as to wheat. There is a great similarity between wheat and rye and many who are allergic to wheat are also allergic to rye.

Boiled dressings
Bouillons
Breads*
Cakes, candy, and cookies*
Creamed pies
Doughnuts, glazed rolls
Egg dishes in all forms
French toast
Hollandaise sauce
Ice cream
Macaroni and spaghetti*
Malted drinks
Marshmallows
Mayonnaise*
Meat loaf*
Noodles*
Ready-mix cakes and puddings
Sausages
Tartar sauce

Foods Allowed

All meats and vegetables
Crackers
Fish—so long as egg is not used if it's breaded
Gingersnaps
Potatoes and rice
Poultry

THE MILK-FREE DIET

Milk allergies are widespread—often the result, some believe, of bottle feeding babies. People whose heritage does not include milk-drinking—blacks and American Indians, for instance—frequently find themselves sensitive to milk. Generally, this sensitivity is to milk sugar and usually produces diarrhea. It is different from a true allergy to milk protein. Sometimes a milk allergy manifests itself after a person develops an ulcer and is ordered to drink a lot of milk. Commonly this has to do with milk sugar and is different from a true allergy to milk protein.

While cow's milk and goat's milk contain the same casein fraction, there is a second protein fraction, called lactalbumin, which is different in cow's and goat's milk. This may be why some people can drink goat's milk with safety, although they are allergic to cow's milk. An allergy to cow's milk does not necessarily mean that one will be allergic to all cheese made with cow's milk, and a cheese allergy may result from other factors than milk. The following list indicates some of the products containing cow's milk. A star * indicates that there are some milk-free brands, or varieties, available and you can create your own substitutes at home, choosing milk other than cow's milk.

Foods to Avoid

Baking powder biscuits
Bread*
Bologna
Butter
Cakes*
Cheeses*
Chowders
Creamed foods and sauces
Custards
Doughnuts
Ice cream
Puddings

Foods Allowed

Beverages: cocoa made with water
           coffee and tea free of milk or cream
           fruit and vegetable juices
Breads made without milk
Cakes made without milk
Cereals eaten with fruit or juices or plain
Cookies made without milk
Cornmeal muffins
Crackers and biscuits made without milk
Fish, meat, and poultry
Fruit and vegetables

THE CORN-FREE DIET

Some allergists believe that corn is today's No. 1 allergen-producing food, the result of the great increase in the use of corn as an ingredient. Sugar from corn can produce allergic reactions in some while sugar from beet and cane do not. While some people can tolerate corn in one form and not another—it has been demonstrated that some people can have an allergic reaction to cornmeal mush or muffins, for instance, and yet not be bothered by fresh corn at all—a corn allergy suggests caution in using any product containing corn. For example, while very little of the corn antigen may remain in corn oil, a person highly sensitive to corn can suffer a reaction from eating a salad with a corn oil dressing or a chicken fried in corn oil.

If a severe reaction to corn is evidenced during the elimination diet, it is best to test out individual products before adding them to a basic diet.

The following list of products containing corn is incomplete. Check labels. Foods followed by asterisk * indicates some corn-free types are available.

Foods to Avoid

Bacon
Baking mixes: biscuits, doughnuts, pancakes, pie crusts
Baking powder*
Batters for fish, fowl, meat
Beer and ale
Cakes, candy
Catsup
Cereals
Cheeses
Chili
Chop suey
Custards, cream pies, cream puffs
Flour*
French dressing
Frozen vegetables
Fruit juices
Fruits—canned, frozen
Gelatin capsules
Gelatin desserts
Gin, whiskey

Graham crackers
Grape juice
Gravies
Hams
Ice creams
Oleomargarine
Peanut butter*
Powdered sugar
Rice (coated)
Salad dressings*
Sandwich spreads
Sauces for meats, fish, sundaes, vegetables
Soy bean milk
String beans—canned, frozen
Tortillas
Wine, American*
Corn is also in:
Aspirin
Bath powder
Body powders
Chewing gum
Gummed papers: envelopes, labels, stamps, stickers, tapes
Popcorn
Starch
Talcum powders

ASPIRIN-CONTAINING COMPOUNDS

Aspirin has been implicated as a specific in causing asthma attacks. Aspirin is used as an ingredient in a great many drugs sold over the counter. The list below is incomplete. If in doubt, ask your pharmacist.

Acetylsalicylic Acid
Alka-Seltzer
Amgesic Tablets
Amytal and Aspirin Pulvules
Anacin
Anahist
A.P.C. Tablets

A.P.C. with Demerol
A.S.A. Enseals and Pulvules and Suppositories
Aspirin Aluminun (chewable)
Aspirin Compound Capsules and Tablets
Aspirin Dulcets and Supprettes
Aspirin Tablets
Bufferin
Coricidin
Daprisal
Darvon
Dristan
Empirin
Emprazil Tablets
Equagesic Tablets
Excedrin
Fiorinal
4-Way Cold Tablets
Midol
Multihist A.P.C. Capsules
Novahistine A.P.C. Capsules
Novrad with A.S.A. Capsules
P.A.C. Capsules and Tablets
Percodan
Phenaphen Capsules
Phensal Capsules and Tablets
Robaxisal Tablets
Tetrex-A.P.C. with Bristamin
Thephorin A-C Tablets
Zactirin Tablets

Resource List

Encasings for mattresses and box springs:

Allergen-Proof Encasings
P.O. Box 03221
Dept. JA
Cleveland, Ohio 44117

Allergen-Proof Encasings
325 Devonshire
Windsor, Ontario, Canada

Allergy-Free Products for the Home
1162 West Lynn
Springfield, Missouri 05802

Sprays to rid basements of mold:

Captan, available from gardeners' or farmers' supply stores. Captan spraying must be done with pressure spraying equipment and the room must be closed for 2–5 hours until the mist settles.

Expanded breathing exercises (illustrated)

"Breathing Exercises for Asthmatic Children"
American Academy of Pediatrics
P.O. Box 1034
Evanston, Illinois 60204

"Exercises for Asthma and Emphysema"
Asthma Research Council
28, Norfolk Place
London, W.E.
England
Price: $1.00, postage free.

Glossary

ADRENAL—adjacent to the kidneys; specifically, relating to or derived from the adrenal glands.

ADRENAL GLANDS—a pair of complex endocrine glands located at the upper poles of the kidneys. Epinephrine, or the hormone adrenalin, is produced by specialized cells in the center of the glands while the outer shell forms several hormones significant in control of salt and water balance, sugar metabolism, and other body reactions. These hormones are called steroids and are related to or identified with cortisone.

ADRENALIN—trademark for a preparation of epinephrine.

ADRENERGEN—a drug having a physiological action resembling that of adrenalin.

ADRENERGIC—liberating adrenalin or a substance like adrenalin; activated by adrenalin.

ADRENOCORTICAL—of, belonging to, or derived from the cortex or outer shell of the adrenal glands.

AEROSOL—suspension of solid or liquid particles in air or gas; a substance and a propellant in a container with a valve through which the substance is dispensed.

AIR SACS—element of the lungs, each of which is subdivided into five or six alveoli, which are very minute structures with extremely thin walls.

ALLERGEN—a substance that induces allergy; an antigen to which one is allergic.

ALLERGIST—a medical doctor specializing in the treatment of allergies.

ALLERGY—a pathological reaction (marked by sneezing, or respiratory problem and asthma attack, or itching and skin rashes, or other responses) to certain foods, drugs, inhalants, or other substances. Viruses and parasites also can cause allergic reactions.

ALVEOLI—air cells of the lungs. The lungs contain an estimated 750,000,000 alveoli. They impart a spongy texture to the lungs.

AMINOPHYLLIN—a drug inducing bronchodilation.

AMP—cyclic chemical substance. (See *GMP*.)

ANAPHYLACTIC REACTION—an acute allergic reaction producing a variety of symptoms up to and including shock or even death.

ANATOMY—the structural makeup of an organism or any of its parts.

ANTIBACTERIAL—inimical to bacteria.

ANTIBIOTIC—a substance produced by a microorganism (as a bacterium or a fungus) or manufactured by chemical synthesis. In dilute solution it has the capacity to inhibit the growth of, or kill, microorganisms (such as a disease germ).

ANTIBODY—any of various globulins normally present in the body or produced in response to infection or by administration of suitable antigens or haptens, that combine specifically with antigens (toxins, bacteria, or foreign red-blood cells) to neutralize them.

ANTIGEN—a protein or carbohydrate substance (such as a toxin, enzyme, or any of certain constituents of blood corpuscles or of cells) that, when introduced into the body, stimulates production of an antibody. Not all antigens induce allergy.

ANTIHISTAMINE—any of various compounds used for treating allergic reactions by inhibiting formation of or neutralizing histamine.

AORTA—the chief arterial trunk of the body that carries blood from the heart to be distributed to all parts of the body.

AUTOGENOUS VACCINE—a vaccine prepared from cultures obtained from a specific lesion of the patient and used to immunize the patient against further spread and progress of the same organism.

AUTONOMIC—acting independently; for example, the autonomic nervous system.

AUTONOMIC NERVOUS SYSTEM—the part of the nervous system that innervates smooth and cardiac muscles and glandular tissues; that governs actions which are more or less autonomic (such as secretion, digestion, respiration, heart, and circulation); and that consists of the sympathetic nervous system and parasympathetic nervous system.

BACTERIA—plural of bacterium; commonly refers to organisms which produce infection in man.

BIOLOGY—the science of life; a branch of knowledge that deals with living organisms and vital processes.

BRAND NAME—trademarked name identifying a specific product.

BRONCHI—plural of bronchus.

BRONCHIAL—relating to, or associated with, the bronchi or their ramifications in the lungs.

BRONCHIAL ARTERY—any branch of the descending aorta or first intercostal artery that accompanies the bronchi.

BRONCHIAL ASTHMA—asthma resulting from spasmodic contraction of bronchial muscles, constriction of the bronchi, and accumulation of mucus in the respiratory passages.

BRONCHIAL GLAND—any of the lymphatic glands situated at the branching of the trachea and along the bronchi.

BRONCHIAL TREE—the bronchi together with their branches.

BRONCHIAL TUBES—a bronchus and any of its branches.

BRONCHIAL VEIN—any vein accompanying the bronchi and their branches.

BRONCHIECTASIS—a chronic inflammatory or degenerative condition of one or more bronchi or bronchioles, marked by dilation and loss of elasticity of the walls.

BRONCHIOLE—a minute, thin-walled branch of a bronchus, that terminates in one or more pulmonary alveoli.

BRONCHIOLITIS—any inflammation of the bronchioles.

BRONCHITIS—any inflammation of the bronchial tubes.

BRONCHODILATOR—any drug that causes relaxation of bronchial muscles, resulting in expansion of the air passages of the bronchi.

BRONCHOSPASM—constriction of the air passages of the lungs by spasmodic contraction of the bronchial muscles.

BRONCHOSPIROMETRY—independent measurement of the vital capacity of each lung by means of an instrument called a spirometer in direct continuity with one of the primary bronchi.

BRONCHUS—either of the two primary divisions of the trachea that lead respectively into the right and the left lung and their large branches. They are structurally similar to the trachea.

CAPILLARIES—tiny blood vessels derived from small arteries.

CARBOHYDRATES—one of the six essential nutrients. Sugar is an example.

CARBON DIOXIDE—a by-product of body metabolism which is expelled from the body through the lungs.

CAROTID—either of the two main arteries that supply blood to the head.

CELLULAR METABOLISM—the vital processes of a cell. Cellular metabolism consists of respiration (oxygen-carbon dioxide exchange), the burning of food for energy, and the formation of waste products; the means by which the cell sustains its own life and obtains energy to carry on its functions.

CELLULAR REACTION—reaction in the cells to a wide variety of occurrences, such as a nervous stimulus, receipt of oxygen or a chemical, etc.

CHEMORECEPTOR—any sense or organ responding to a chemical stimulus (such as a smell or taste receptor or one of the carotid receptors that react to changes in the chemical composition of the blood).

CONSTRICTION—the act of drawing together or tightening.

CONTINUOUS BRONCHODILATION—the goal of consistent administration of bronchodilating drugs, the objective being twenty-four-hour-a-day easy breathing through relaxed air passages.

CONTRAINDICATION—a term applied, ordinarily, to reasons why a drug should not be prescribed or administered to a particular person. Relative contraindication means that the potential dangers must be weighed against immediate needs and potential benefit from the drug in question.

CORTISONE—a hormone produced by the adrenal cortex, which regulates sodium retention. Medically, it can be isolated and purified from the adrenal glands of certain domesticated animals but more usually it is produced chemically. It may effect carbohydrate metabolism. It is used in asthma treatment, generally in form of pills, injections, or sprays. It is also used in treatment of rheumatoid arthritis and other diseases.

CROMOLYN SODIUM—generic name for a new group of drugs used in asthma treatment under the brand names of Aarane and Intal.

CULTURE—cultivation of living material (bacteria or tissue).

DIAPHRAGM—thin sheet of muscle and connective tissue separating the chest and abdominal cavities.

DILATION—spreading apart or opening.

ELIMINATION DIET—diet restricted to a few normally non-allergic foods, followed by testing of individual foods one at a time.

EMPHYSEMA—a degenerative disease characterized by decreased lung elasticity. The capacity of the lungs to absorb oxygen is greatly reduced. The lung air sacs are overdistended and often ruptured. The residual air is greatly increased.

EPHEDRINE—a white crystalline alkaloid used in the treatment of asthma, hay fever, and nasal congestion. It stimulates the sympathetic nervous system to produce bronchodilation.

EPINEPHRINE—a colorless crystalline compound used as a bronchodilator in the treatment of asthma. Synonymous with adrenalin.

ESSENTIAL NUTRIENTS—elements needed for sound nutrition (protein, carbohydrates, fats, vitamins, minerals, water).

EXHALE—expel air from the lungs; breathe out.

EXPIRATION—the action or process of releasing air from the lungs through the nose or mouth; the escape of carbon dioxide from the body protoplasm through the blood or lungs or by diffusion.

EXTRINSIC ASTHMA—asthma caused from outside agents, such as weather, inhalants, etc. (See *intrinsic asthma*.)

GENERIC—relating to or descriptive of a group or class of medicines available for common use; not protected by a trademark. A single generic drug may have many brand names.

GENETICS—the science of heredity.

GLOBULINS—any of a class of simple proteins that are characterized by their almost complete insolubility in pure water and by their solubility in dilute salt solutions that are coagulable by heat and that occur widely in plant and animal tissues (such as blood plasma or serum).

GMP—a cyclic chemical substance, which works in a seesaw fashion with a cyclic chemical substance labeled AMP. The elements which favor a balance of GMP will have a particularly adverse effect and produce inflammatory agents from specific cells which are likely to cause asthma. (See *AMP*.)

HAY FEVER—an acute allergic nasal catarrh that is sometimes accompanied by asthma or asthmatic symptoms.

HEREDITARY—genetically transmitted or capable of being genetically transmitted from parent to offspring.

HEREDITY—the sum of the qualities and potentialities of a person that are genetically derived from his ancestors; the germinal constitution of an individual.

HISTAMINASE—an enzyme produced in the liver and intestines capable of destroying histamine.

HISTAMINE—a substance derived from the breakdown of histidine in body tissues. Normally present throughout the body in minute amounts, in larger amounts it causes symptoms often associated with allergies. Histamine reactions may be generalized, as in hay fever, or may be localized, as in insect bites and stings.

HORMONE—a specific organic product of living cells that, transported by body fluids, produces a specific effect on cells remote from its point of origin; a product exerting a stimulatory or excitatory effect on a cellular activity without participating in that activity.

INDICATION—reasons for doing a specific thing, such as for taking a particular drug.

INFECTION—the state produced by the establishment of an infective agent in or on a suitable host; an infective agent (as a fungus, bacterium, or virus).

INHALE—to draw in by breathing; to breathe in.

INNERVATE—to supply with nerves; to arouse or stimulate (a nerve or an organ) to activity.

INSPIRATION—the act of drawing air into the lungs.

INTRAVENOUS INJECTION—an injection administered by needle into the veins. In acute asthma attack, aminophyllin is often administered intravenously.

INTRINSIC ASTHMA—asthma having causes other than allergies; for example, respiratory or other infections, such as sinus infections. It is non-seasonal. (See *extrinsic asthma*.)

MAST CELL—a cell contained in many tissues, including the lungs, which can release certain granules, especially on stimulation. In the asthmatic these granules may be provoked by triggers to release chemical substances, including histamine, which cause bronchospasm.

METABOLISM—the chemical changes in living cells by which energy is provided for vital processes and activities.

MIXED ASTHMA—where the causes are both extrinsic (allergies) and intrinsic (infection).

MUCUS—a viscid, slippery secretion that is produced by glands and that serves to moisten and protect membranes; in asthma attacks it can be variously fluffy white, nearly colorless, or yellowish or greenish. Sometimes, in a severe attack, it can produce plugs or strings of thickened material.

NEGATIVE SKIN TEST—where injection of a substance under the skin does not evoke a raised red bump or wheal, thus demonstrating to the allergist that the person is not allergic to that substance.

PARASYMPATHETIC NERVOUS SYSTEM—the part of the autonomic nervous system that tends to work in opposite fashion to the sympathetic nerves. (See *sympathetic nervous system.*)

PATHOLOGIC PHYSIOLOGY—alterations of function which take place when abnormalities exist.

PERENNIAL—occurring through all seasons.

PNEUMONIA—infection of the lung tissue.

PREDISPOSITION—a condition of being predisposed; inclination, tendency.

PREDNISOLONE—a cortisone compound similar in action to prednisone.

PREDNISONE—a crystalline or amorphous glucocorticoid drug that is an analogue of cortisone and is used similarly to cortisone.

PROSTAGLANDINS—a substance found in tissues, deriving its name from its initial identification in the testicles of sheep but since found in the tissues of many organs, including the lungs.

PULMONARY—relating to the lungs.

PULMONARY ARTERY—an artery that conveys venous blood from the heart to the lungs.

RALES—crackles, wheezes, or other adventitious sounds heard when air passes through a narrowed passage or one containing moisture.

RESIDUAL AIR—"stale air" in the lungs not expelled after deep breathing.

RESPIRATION—a single complete act of breathing; it supplies oxygen needed by the cells for metabolism and relieves them of the carbon dioxide formed in energy-producing reactions.

RESPIRATORY CENTER—a group of cells in the brain, which direct the mechanism of breathing.

SIDE-EFFECTS—undesirable conditions that can arise from overdosage with one or more drugs.

SPASM—a sudden constriction or tightening.

SPUTUM—matter discharged from air passages in diseases of the lungs, bronchi, or upper respiratory tract that contains mucus and sometimes pus, bacterial products, and other material.

SPUTUM CULTURE—test to determine precise contents of sputum.

SRS-A—a slow reacting substance of anaphylaxis

STALE AIR—see *residual air*.

STEROID—any of a class of compounds characterized by a polycyclic structure.

SUPPOSITORY—a solid preparation made usually of medicated cocoa butter or glycerinated gelatin. It is usually in the form of a cylinder for introduction into the rectum where it melts at body temperature to release medication.

SYMPATHETIC NERVOUS SYSTEM—the part of the autonomic nervous system that contains chiefly adrenergic fibers and that tends to depress secretion, dilate bronchi, and cause the contraction of blood vessels.

SYMPTOM—subjective evidence of disease or physical disturbance observed by the person; something that indicates the existence of something else.

THORACIC CAVITY—the body cavity lying above the diaphragm, bounded peripherally by the wall of the chest and containing the heart and the lungs.

TIMED VITAL CAPACITY—the amount of air expired in one second.

TOXIN—any of various poisonous substances that are specific products of the metabolic activities of living organisms; colloidal substances related to proteins and usually very unstable.

TRACHEA—the main trunk of the system of tubes by which air passes to and from the lungs.

TRIGGERS—atmospheric, physical, or chemical conditions, states, or substances liable to initiate an asthmatic attack in a person predisposed to asthma.

VITAL CAPACITY—the amount of air brought into the lungs and expelled in one respiration.

Index